In memory of my mother and my dog Ooey

Special thanks to my father, Ted, Dr. Blair Bethel, the Neffs, and Peggy and Rick.

I would also like to thank my staff, clients and patients who have inspired me to share this information.

ABOUT THE AUTHOR

Dr. Shearer owns and operates a small animal veterinary practice in Columbus, Ohio. In addition, she is a university guest lecturer and makes frequent appearances on local television as a veterinary advisor. She manages the Pet Education Center that promotes pet health care through education, and she teaches pet first-aid classes and pet geriatric classes at the Center. Dr. Shearer is a regular guest veterinary advisor on a radio show for the blind.

Dr. Shearer has started a number of local neighborhood programs to promote animal welfare, including the Rusty Ranger Club (to encourage children to be kind to animals) and a lost pet block-watch program. She is the author of two other books: *Emergency First Aid For Your Dog* and *Emergency First Aid For Your Cat.* Dr. Shearer is a member of the American Veterinary Medical Association, the Ohio Veterinary Medical Association, the Veterinary Laser Association, and the American Society for Laser Medicine and Surgery. She is licensed to practice in Ohio and California. She is one of the few veterinarians who still make house calls.

In her spare time, Dr. Shearer cares for her two horses, five pigs, ten dogs and six cats.

PROLOGUE

On January 12, 1995, at 10:00 pm I said my last good-bye to an old friend. Ooey had seen me through many life changes. He gave me companionship during my undergraduate and veterinary school days, and when I began practicing veterinary medicine, he watched my career progress. During all those years, he asked very little while he gave me unconditional love and support.

I worked hard to make Ooey's life comfortable, but his last year proved a real challenge, when his aging problems took their toll. We shared a great deal during his final months, and I learned through trial and error how to keep an old dog comfortable. Since then, I have made it my mission to collect and share as much information as possible on the needs of aging dogs.

TABLE OF CONTENTS

PROLOGUE

PART 1 - FIRST THINGS FIRST FOR DOGS OVER FIVE

PART 2 - DISEASE PREVENTION AND EARLY DETECTION

PART 3 - PHYSICAL PROBLEMS

PART 4 - CREATIVE IDEAS TO COPE WITH THE PROBLEMS OF AGING

PART 5 - TREATMENT OPTIONS

PART 6 - ANESTHESIA AND SURGERY

PART 7 - FINAL DECISIONS AND COPING WITH LOSS

APPENDICES

BIBLIOGRAPHY / 245

INDEX / 247

PART 1

FIRST THINGS FIRST FOR

DOGS OVER FIVE

SPECIAL COMMENTS

This book is a guide for keeping your dog healthy and comfortable during the middle and later years, which begins at approximately five years of age. This book will provide you with a foundation of practical knowledge and creative solutions so that you can make informed decisions regarding your dog's care when, or even before, your dog shows signs of having special needs.

This book should be used as a supplement to, not a substitute for, proper veterinary care. Because your veterinarian will be able to advise you best based on the particular circumstances of your dog's life changes, you should contact your veterinarian for additional advice appropriate for your dog.

INTRODUCTION

A dog over five years of age needs special care to be kept safe, comfortable, and healthy. At times, you may not be aware when your dog becomes more dependent upon you, and not providing proper care may compromise the dog's health and comfort. The special care required by a dog over five includes additional attention, increased medical care, and/or an adjustment of lifestyle. Your additional responsibility in caring for your dog usually comes easily because of the bonding that occurs over the years.

Regardless of whether your dog is in good health, many changes occur with aging, some subtle and others more obvious. By learning now what these changes are, how to identify them and how to prevent or treat them, you will be better prepared to care for your dog through the years; you will be able to provide your "best friend" with the appropriate comforts and care as the needs arise. By reading this book, you will learn at least fifty precautions that you might take to provide for your dog's well-being, plus you will learn to identify and care for the stresses of aging. You will learn to recognize the top ten warning signs of early illness, as well as the ten signs of cancer. In addition, you will learn the basics of how to identify and respond to your dog's needs.

As the table of contents for this book indicates, there is a multitude of topics that need to be addressed regarding proper care for dogs over five. This book provides basic and creative solutions to a variety of aging problems and offers specific information regarding a wide range of conditions, symptoms, diagnoses and treatments. After reading this book, you should be better able to make informed decisions regarding everything from daily routines to preventive care to medical treatments, and you should be able to develop an appropriate health plan and exercise plan for your dog. You will learn basic as well as creative solutions to difficulties ranging from arthritis to weight loss (or gain). You will learn methods of early detection for major illnesses, such as cancer, plus you will be taught techniques for making your pet comfortable in a variety of situations. After reading this book, you should be able to recognize the symptoms of specific problems, as well as have a knowledge about their diagnosis and treatment. You will be able to make educated decisions about your dog's treatment options regarding matters such as hospitalization versus outpatient treatment for a medical problem, and decisions regarding surgeries, anesthetics and alternative treatments.

ACCESS TO HOME AND VETERINARY CARE

Providing access to continual home and veterinary care is important for aging dogs because of their increased risk for disease and their decreased ability to adjust to change.

One of the important aspects of providing care is to make sure your dog can be identified if lost. Even when dogs are kept mostly inside or in a secured yard, they are often masters of escape. Older dogs get confused easily and may wander from home. With decreased senses, they may lack the ability to find their way back. Therefore, all dogs should be provided with an identification tag. The tag should include the owner's name, address, and telephone number on one side and the veterinarian's name, address and telephone number on the opposite side. Proper identification is important in facilitating treatment. If a pet is away from its home and suffers an illness or injury, the owner can be identified and promptly notified. The identification tag should directly adhere to the pet's collar and should not be left dangling. A dangling tag can become stuck in and on various objects and pose a risk. (However, any identification is better than none.) Ask your veterinarian about a break-away safety collar for your dog. Also, make sure that your dog's collar is not too tight; you should be able to fit two fingers easily between the collar and the dog's neck. If your dog is gaining weight, check the collar every week to make sure the pet has not outgrown it. If your dog is losing weight, tighten the collar so that it is not too loose.

In addition to an identification tag, you may wish to consider a form of permanent marking to ensure that your dog can be identified if its tags are accidentally or intentionally removed. Permanent marking includes a tattoo or a subcutaneous implant. The subcutaneous implant is a microchip with an identification number. It is inserted under the skin of the shoulder area. It is about the size of a piece of rice and is implanted by injection. All shelters and most veterinary hospitals scan lost dogs to check for these chips. The transponder transmits a number which is registered with the American Kennel Club; the number can be traced 24 hours a day so that the dog's owner or veterinarian can be contacted. If your dog is lost or stolen, these permanent markings will enable you to positively identify the pet as belonging to you, and a permanent marking should alert anyone who comes into contact with the pet that the dog is not an unwanted stray. Ask your veterinarian for more details about these methods of identification.

Besides good identification, make arrangements to have access to veterinary care 24 hours a day. This may take some planning, especially if you live in a rural area. Most large cities have pet emergency-care centers. Even though the pet may have a regular veterinarian, it is a good idea to have at least one other doctor available as a backup during the day. Also, make arrangements to have two night-time veterinarians available. The veterinarians' telephone numbers should be listed near the phone.

A first-aid kit should be prepared and readily available for use if needed in a crisis. This insures continuity in care between the home and hospital. The most important feature of a first-aid kit is accessibility; the kit must be available when a problem arises. See Appendix I for a list of items found in a dog's first-aid kit.

Arrangements should be prepared ahead of time if you have to be away from your dog. A home pet sitter should be considered over a boarding kennel for aging dogs. Some dogs fear separation from their owners and their home. A dog's stress level can be lessened by a comfortable, familiar environment. The pet sitter should know whom to contact in case of an emergency. The dog's veterinarian should also be notified of treatment preferences in the event of an emergency when the owner is unavailable; otherwise the veterinarian will likely provide only basic care until given permission to proceed with additional treatments.

By following these suggestions, you can provide your dog with continual home care and veterinary care when needed.

FIFTY COMMON-SENSE PRECAUTIONS

Even though dogs over five are usually not as active as younger ones, they still have a tendency to find trouble. In addition, some dogs over five will need extra supervision due to medical conditions and/or age-related factors.

As dogs grow older, they may get confused more easily. Older dogs often have diminished senses, such as loss of hearing and/or decreased vision, and they do not have the reflexes of younger dogs. Considering the number of hazards that exist outdoors, older dogs should ideally be confined to the house or kept in a secured yard. Older dogs that are permitted to roam outdoors might explore places that are dangerous for them, and when they do get into trouble, you might not be there to help. Also, with unconfined dogs, it is difficult to monitor attitude, appetite, toilet habits and other behavior for signs of illness; many seriously ill or injured dogs that are not confined seek hiding places and often die.

Dogs that spend most of their time outside unconfined have more exposure than confined dogs to poisons and a greater risk of traumas from cars, guns, other animals and even people. Because trapping is a cool-weather sport, in the winter months your dog should never be permitted to roam in any area where trapping may occur. Wooded areas, especially near creek beds, are common places for leg-hold traps to be set. In addition, dogs that are permitted to roam can pose a threat to people and other people's pets. Unconfined dogs, especially older or debilitated dogs, also have a higher risk of contracting infections because of their increased exposure to disease. Infections such as canine distemper, parainfluenza, leptospirosis, hepatitis, parvovirus, coronavirus, bordetella and rabies virus can be fatal. Parasitic infections can also cause serious disease.

During colder months, older dogs that exhibit aging changes should be kept indoors or in a comfortable garage, barn, or shed with a heat source. If the dog cannot be kept inside the house or other heated structure, it should at least have good shelter away from drafts and dampness. The shelter (i.e., dog house) should be just big enough for the dog to lie down and to stand. Too much height, depth

15

and length does not promote heat conservation. The shelter should contain clean, dry bedding, ideally straw. Wet or soiled bedding must be replaced immediately. When the temperature falls below freezing, your pet should be moved inside or provided with an alternative heat source, such as a heat lamp. Your dog's paws should be kept clean of ice, salt and mud. Also, always provide your dog with fresh food and water. (Note that water may freeze quickly in the winter months.)

In the summer months, if your dog is outdoors, access to plenty of fresh water is especially important. If your dog sometimes tips over its water bowl, partially bury the bowl in the ground. Make sure your pet has adequate shade from summer midday heat. If your dog spends time in a shed or garage, good ventilation is essential. Older dogs often are not able to regulate body temperature as well as younger dogs, and older dogs are therefore more likely to suffer heat stroke or dehydration. In warmer weather, preexisting disease also makes an older dog more prone to heat stroke.

Because dogs have a tendency to eat grass, it is important to keep your dog indoors if your lawn has been chemically treated recently with pesticides or fertilizers. Lawn chemicals can poison a dog or may cause chemical burns to the pet's feet. Also, if you have recently sprayed insecticides inside your home, keep your dog out of the rooms that have been sprayed until the chemicals dissipate. An older dog may not have the same tolerance for chemicals as a younger dog because a dog's liver, which serves as a filter, may tend to function less effectively as a dog ages.

Even indoors, dogs are not without risk, but modifying the home environment can help decrease the likelihood of problems. Dog-proof your home by removing potential hazards. Secure all medications, household cleaners and other potential toxins in drawers or cabinets out of reach of your pet. Remove any choke hazards and be aware of everyday items that can cause choking. For example, make sure any bones from an evening meal are immediately discarded, and make sure that any toys, rawhide bones, etc. cannot become choke hazards. Make sure electrical and other cords are not dangling in a manner that will entice your dog to chew on them. Electrical cords can cause severe burns or death if your dog chews through the protective insulation, and any type of cord (e.g., telephone, drapery, etc.) poses a danger of strangulation. Also, keep your dog's toenails well-trimmed to prevent them from catching on carpets and furniture. Overgrown toenails can cause lameness or complicate arthritis in an older dog. If your dog has any difficulty with its balance, block stairways to prevent the dog from accidentally falling.

When your dog is in your home, keep all windows at least partially closed to prevent your pet from accidentally or intentionally using a window as a door. Note that screens in windows may not be enough of a barrier to prevent your dog from falling or jumping through a window. This especially poses a hazard for older dogs suffering from separation anxiety or fearing thunderstorms.

While some older dogs enjoy toys, make sure that any toy you give to your dog is constructed so that your dog cannot eat portions that may be nondigestible. If portions are missing, remove and replace the toy. No toys should have any strings dangling because ingested string can cut through a dog's digestive tract. All toys should be large enough and strong enough that neither the whole toy nor any part of it can be swallowed. Socks, hose and shoes with laces are also choking hazards and should be kept out of your dog's reach.

Dogs have a keen sense of smell, and ordinary household items can become hazards if they contain food smells. For example, a steel wool pad that you have used to scrub a pan after cooking bacon or some other meat can become a deadly enticement for your pet. Dogs will sometimes eat knives, forks and other utensils used to prepare foods. Even flavored dental floss is appetizing to some dogs, and dental floss may cause fatal bowel injuries if swallowed. Aluminum foil or any other wrap that has been used on any food product that might be appealing to your dog should be discarded in a manner that prevents your dog from having access to it. You should note that metal products like steel wool pads and aluminum foil are particularly destructive to a dog's digestive system. Similarly, Christmas-tree tinsel is extremely destructive to a dog's stomach and bowels, and you should never decorate a Christmas tree with tinsel if your dog has any chance of getting to the tree.

Toxic indoor plants should be identified and removed, or kept out of reach. (Refer to the book *Emergency First-Aid for Your Dog* by Dr. Tamara Shearer for an extensive list of poisonous plants, their side effects, and their treatments.) If your dog is permitted outside, you should attempt to limit its access to potentially harmful plants.

Never use a flea product on a dog that is debilitated or appears to be ill, unless instructed by your veterinarian. Flea products for dogs can become toxic even when used properly. Always read and follow product labels carefully because improper use can be extremely hazardous to your dog's health.

Never feed your dog chocolate, table scraps or bones. Chocolate is poisonous to dogs because it contains theobromine, which they cannot metabolize. In general, table scraps can predispose a dog to pancreatitis and other digestive upsets, and milk can be a major cause of diarrhea. Older dogs seem to be more sensitive to changes in diet and are especially prone to pancreatitis and colitis. Bones cannot be digested and can pierce the lining of the digestive tract, possibly causing fatal peritonitis (inflammation within the abdomen). As a preventive measure, keep all people food away from your dog, and keep trash containers secured.

Older dogs may suffer from arthritis pain. Do not attempt to alleviate your dog's pain with your own medications. People medications are often poisonous to dogs. Acetaminophen (Tylenol®) and ibuprofen (Advil®) are frequently fatal for dogs, even in small doses. Never administer medications of any type without specific instructions from your veterinarian.

Dogs suffering from arthritis may benefit from an exercise program that includes swimming as a substitute for running. Swimming is easier on a dog's joints yet provides the same cardiovascular and muscle benefits. However, it is important to note that the risk of drowning increases with age due to medically-related problems such as heart failure, arthritis and decreased stamina. Make sure you supervise your dog's swimming, and use common sense regarding safe swimming conditions. You might consider obtaining a life vest for your dog. If the surf is high or the current is swift, keep your dog out of the water. Also, make sure your dog has easy access to land, so that your dog can get out of the water as easily as it gets in.

During transportation, do not allow your dog to ride on your lap, stand on the back window ledge or engage in any behavior that might detract from your attention to your driving or put the pet at additional risk in the event of an accident. Do not permit your dog to put its entire head out of the window; the wind from the moving car blows debris that can injure a dog's eyes. Also, never transport a dog in the back of an open pickup truck. Older dogs may have poor balance and coordination so provide a safer traveling environment by using a pet carrier or a pet safety belt, or a leash attached to the seat. You might also consider padding the floor with blankets in case your dog falls out of the seat. When you are driving, pay careful attention to accelerate and stop smoothly and gently to help your dog's balance. Also, if your car has a passenger-side air bag, keep your dog in the back seat to prevent severe injury or death.

Finally, make sure your dog is up-to-date on its vaccinations. In addition to vaccinations, there are preventive medications that your dog may need. For example, heartworm disease, which is spread by mosquitoes, can be prevented by monthly medications. The section on Preventive Health Care lists the vaccinations and medications that your dog should receive as well as a timetable for vaccinations and boosters and medications. You should note that many dog diseases that are easily preventable with a vaccine are often fatal, including rabies, which can be transmitted to people.

Taking reasonable precautions, discussed above and listed below, should decrease the risk of a problem, regardless of your dog's age or condition. Following these precautions may save your dog's life.

---

1. Keep telephone cords, drapery cords and electrical cords out of reach.
2. Do not decorate a Christmas tree with tinsel.
3. Keep all utensils, foils, wraps, scrub pads, etc. that may contain food smells out of reach of your dog.
4. Keep windows above the ground floor at least partially closed.
5. Always supervise a dog that is swimming.
6. Honk your car horn before pulling out of the driveway.
7. Never call your dog to come if the dog has to cross a road in front of cars. Instead, cross the street yourself, and then bring the dog to the other side with you.
8. Never allow your dog to ride with its head outside the car window.
9. Never allow your dog to ride in the back of an open pick-up truck.
10. Prepare a first-aid kit for emergencies. (See Appendix I.)
11. Provide good ventilation during hot summer months.
12. Never leave a dog alone in a hot car with the windows up.
13. Never leave a dog alone for an extended period of time.
14. When your dog is outside unsupervised, keep the pet in a secured area (i.e., secured with a fence or an invisible fence) or keep the dog tied.
15. Keep the dog indoors if the pet's age and condition necessitate extra security.
16. Provide your dog with an identification tag.
17. In the winter, provide fresh water, and change it before it freezes.

18. In cool months, provide dry, draft-free shelter. The shelter should be just big enough for the dog to lie down and to stand; too much height, depth and length does not promote heat conservation and will not serve well as a shelter. Put bedding (i.e., clean, dry straw) in the shelter.

19. During hot summer months, provide well-ventilated shelter and extra drinking water.

20. Never withhold water from an older dog without the advice of your veterinarian.

21. Do not overfeed your dog (i.e., do not let your dog gain excess weight).

22. Never feed cat food to your dog. Cat food lacks the balance of nutrients essential for healthy dogs. Also, it may cause diarrhea, or the high fat content may promote obesity.

23. Never give milk to your dog. Milk can cause digestive problems, such as diarrhea.

24. Never feed raw fish to your dog. Raw fish causes a thiamine deficiency which may result in loss of appetite, a hunched and painful stance and possibly convulsions. Even if fish is cooked, never feed a dog a diet of fish exclusively.

25. Never feed a dog foods that contain rancid fats or excess polyunsaturated fats because these fats can cause a vitamin E deficiency leading to a variety of muscle diseases.

26. Never feed your dog table scraps, bones or chocolates.

27. Do not supplement a dog's diet without a veterinarian's advice. Wrong supplementation can cause urinary tract problems, metabolic problems and even mineralization of the kidneys.

28. Never oversupplement your dog's diet with vitamin D or fish liver oil. Excess can cause bone disease as well as digestive upset.

29. Keep all trash containers covered, and keep any and all table scraps, especially bones, away from your dog.

30. Make sure that your dog does not have access to socks, hose or shoes/shoelaces.

31. Make sure that all dog toys are sufficiently large and indestructible that they do not pose a risk of choking. Also,

make sure that they do not contain any string or yarn.

32. Identify and remove toxic plants and flowers.
33. Keep your dog off of lawns that have been recently treated with pesticides or fertilizers.
34. Keep your dog out of rooms where you have recently sprayed indoor insecticides.
35. Never use poisonous ant traps.
36. Never use continual-release toilet disinfectants.
37. Properly dispose of antifreeze.
38. Never use snail bait or rat poison.
39. Never give your dog any people medications, such as acetaminophen (Tylenol®) or ibuprofen (Advil®) – these substances can be deadly.
40. Never give any medication without a veterinarian's advice.
41. Keep vaccinations and physical exams up-to-date.
42. Get an annual heartworm test and heartworm preventive medicine.
43. Have the dog's stool checked twice per year for worms.
44. Follow a veterinarian's advice regarding your dog's dental care.
45. Report any problems promptly to your dog's veterinarian.
46. Follow flea-product instructions carefully.
47. Keep paws free of ice, mud and salt; wash and dry the paws.
48. Keep hair coat free of mats (to prevent skin sores).
49. Trim your dog's toenails regularly.
50. Provide regular exercise as advised by your veterinarian.

FINDING A VETERINARIAN

You should not change veterinarians unless there is a good reason. Your usual veterinarian most likely knows your dog well enough to have some insight into your pet's needs. If you do need to find another veterinarian, look for one who is not only knowledgeable but also patient. And make sure the veterinarian listens closely, and communicates well. Because aging dogs may show very subtle changes in health, a veterinarian who takes extra time with your pet may be better able to give advice. The following questions may help you decide if the veterinarian you choose is right for your dog.

I.   Questions to Ask Yourself

A.   Do I feel comfortable with my dog's present veterinarian?

B.   If not, in what areas does the situation not feel
      appropriate? The bedside manner? The communication?
      The doctor's staff? The office hours?

C.   Do I need a doctor who is sympathetic to my needs and feelings
      or am I content with a veterinarian who is technically competent?

D.   Does the staff treat my dog and me with respect and compassion?

II.   Questions to Ask the Veterinarian

A.   *How long is your average office call?*
      A good response would be"as long as it takes." On average, an
      initial examination of a healthy dog should take a minimum of
      30 minutes.

B.   *If I cannot get to you or if my dog is unable to travel, will you
      make a house call?*
      Most veterinarians do not make house calls. Depending upon
      your situation, you may feel a need to have a veterinarian who
      will make a house call.

C.   *What should I do if there is an emergency after hours when your
      office is closed?*
      Your veterinarian should recommend a facility that specializes in

24-hour emergency care. While these facilities are not generally appropriate for routine matters, they tend to have the expertise and specially trained staff to handle critical-care situations. Find out now, before there is an emergency, where the nearest critical-care facility is located and put the phone number in an easily accessible place.

D. *If you are not available, who will take care of my dog? May I meet him or her?*

You should always have a backup veterinarian, and you should make sure you have confidence in the backup. You should always try to meet anyone who might be treating your pet.

E. *Do you allow visitation if my dog becomes hospitalized?*

Many older dogs benefit from family visitation.

F. *Whom do you use or recommend when a situation calls for a second opinion?*

Beware of any doctor who says he or she never needs a second opinion. If the doctor is working in association with another veterinarian at the same facility, ask whether they ever seek outside advice, and if so, under what circumstances. Again, beware of any veterinarian who thinks he or she can always do everything.

G. *Will you tell me what you are going to do with my dog before you do anything, and will you explain any tests you recommend before you run them?*

The answer to both parts of this question should be "yes."

IDENTIFYING STRESSES

Stress and related difficulties are a major problem for aging dogs. In fact, if your dog had a health wish list, the items at the top of the list would probably include: "Keep me free from emotional and physical stress. Provide me proper food and exercise. Give me regular veterinary checkups to identify problems and keep me healthy. Keep me comfortable based on my unique needs." Stress is related to every item on that list, and therefore identifying sources of stress is of paramount importance. Once stresses are identified, solutions can be created to help remedy the situation. The following three lists may be helpful. If you have difficulty answering the questions presented in the third list, consult your veterinarian for guidance.

I. Symptoms of Stress (one or more may be present)

A. Problem behavior (e.g., broken house habits, chewing clothing or furniture, other destructive behavior)

B. Depression

C. Loss of appetite

D. Nervousness

E. Excess excitability

F. Any change in behavior

G. Physical signs (e.g., weight loss, sickly appearance)

II. Typical Causes of Stress

A. Inadequate daily care

    1. Not being let outside frequently enough

    2. Being left alone too often or for too long

    3. Inadequate food and/or water

    4. Inadequate shelter (from heat, cold, rain, etc.)

    5. Inadequate affection

B. Environment
    1. Other dogs or cats, animals or people
    2. Noise
    3. Pollution
    4. Insects and ticks
    5. Any change in environment or change in daily routine
C. Medical
    1. Chronic, untreated conditions
    2. Hereditary defects (e.g., hip dysplasia)
    3. Temporary illness
    4. Arthritis and other age-related conditions

III. Questions to Help Identify Causes of Stress

A. Who might be causing or contributing to the stress?
    1. Is the stress being caused by a family member providing inadequate care (e.g., not letting the dog outside often enough, not providing adequate food, shelter or affection, etc.).
    2. Does the problem lie with health-care providers who are not adequately solving medical problems?
    3. If you have more than one pet, is one of the other pets responsible for, or contributing to, the stress?
B. When, and under what circumstances, do the signs of stress arise?
    1. Are the signs of stress occurring during the day, the night, or all the time?
    2. Is there a pattern to the signs of stress (e.g., worse on weekdays, better after meals, etc.)?
    3. Are the signs of stress new or have they been ongoing?
C. What is the source?
    1. What appears to be the underlying cause of the stress?
    2. What additional causes of stress might be present?
    3. What indicators of stress are present?
    4. If there are behavioral changes, could there be an underlying medical problem?

D. Where is the source?
   1. Is the problem that indicates stress occurring in the house or outside?
   2. Is there a particular room in the house where the problem is worse?
E. Why is there stress?
   1. Is the stress resulting from lack of nursing care at home?
   2. Is the stress due to a medical problem?
   3. Is the stress due to a behavioral change?
F. How can you relieve your pet's stress?
   1. How can you eliminate potential causes of stress?
   2. How can the stress be minimized?
   3. How can you treat underlying problems and conditions?

PART 2

—

DISEASE PREVENTION AND EARLY DETECTION

TOP TEN HEALTH WARNING SIGNS

There are several health warning signs that may appear as a dog ages. Frequently these signs go unnoticed. This section will describe the ten most important changes to watch for as warning signs for potential health problems or disease processes. Note that any change in your dog's behavior or appearance warrants further examination. The purpose of the top ten list, in part, is to make sure that you are familiar with the types of changes to look for and report to your veterinarian.

Loss of appetite is best detected when the dog is fed meals on a schedule and not allowed free access to food throughout the day. A lack of appetite which persists longer than one day should be investigated. It can denote a variety of problems ranging from infection to organ failure. **Weakness** may also denote a variety of problems. Weakness could be a symptom of anemia, organ failure, infection, cancer or diabetes. Even if the weakness resolves on its own, see your veterinarian. **Increased thirst** can be an early warning sign of diabetes, organ failure (especially kidney failure), Cushing's disease, internal bleeding, and some cancers. Except under severe conditions of heat and exercise, a dog should not consume more than one cup of water per day for every seven pounds of body weight. If your dog drinks more than that amount per day, consult your veterinarian. Dogs that start having **broken house habits**, if they are housebroken, may be sending a signal that there is a medical problem. Loss of control over urination and/or bowel movements is a sign of many disease processes, such as urinary irritations or infections, nerve degeneration, hormonal imbalances and a variety of other ailments. Severe or persistent coughing should be investigated by a veterinarian. **Coughing** is the most common sign of heart disease. It may also be a symptom of asthma or bronchitis. If there is a sudden **weight gain or abdominal distension** you should contact your veterinarian as soon as possible. Hormonal imbalances, such as hypothyroidism and Cushing's disease, can cause weight gain. An enlarged abdomen can be caused by a number of problems, including heart failure and the growth of tumors. **Weight loss** should be considered significant when the change in weight is greater than 10% of the average body weight or if other symptoms of illness are noted. Weight loss may be due to a number of changes ranging from worms to cancers. All **lumps and bumps** should be reported to your veterinarian for professional evaluation. Some lumps and bumps may be nothing more than benign cysts, while others may be malignancies. **Vomiting and/or diarrhea** may be a sign of something serious, especially if the symptoms persist. Vomiting and diarrhea may be signs of infection, inflammation, cancers or organ failure. **Bad breath** is a sign that most likely denotes a problem in the mouth or nose. Severe tooth decay, oral and nasal tumors, and infections can cause bad breath. Bad breath should be reported to your veterinarian to avoid any preventable problems.

If any of these signs or any other change is noticed, contact your veterinarian for help. A list of common signs of cancer can be found on page 30. Early recognition of a problem may prevent a more serious situation from occurring and may even save your dog's life.

Top Ten Health Warning Signs
1. Loss of appetite
2. Weakness
3. Increased thirst
4. Broken house habits
5. Coughing
6. Weight gain and/or abdominal distention
7. Weight loss
8. Lumps and Bumps
9. Vomiting and/or diarrhea
10. Bad breath

TEN SIGNS OF CANCER

Dogs over age five are at higher risk of developing cancers. Cancer refers to a group of cells that grow quickly, invade, or spread throughout the body. The different types of cancers may affect any area of the body, ranging from the blood, bone, brain, and breasts to the skin, pancreas, or liver.

Early detection of cancer helps improve the dog's chances of recovery and enables more effective treatments to keep your pet comfortable. If you detect any of these signs in your pet, contact your veterinarian. Much can be done once a dog is diagnosed.

Ten Signs of Cancer
1. Any sore that will not heal
2. Bleeding or discharge from any body opening
3. Abnormal lumps, bumps, growths or swellings that persist, regardless of whether they continue to grow
4. Loss of appetite or difficulty eating or swallowing
5. Weight loss (may or may not be accompanied by loss of appetite)
6. Offensive odor in general or from a particular area
7. Difficulty breathing, loss of energy, weakness or lack of stamina
8. Persistent limping, lameness or stiffness
9. Difficulty urinating or defecating, or increased time required to urinate or defecate
10. A general decline in health, or behavior that seems to indicate rapid aging

SIGNS OF AN EMERGENCY

In addition to the top ten warning signs and the ten signs of cancer, there are some high risk signs that should be recognized as an emergency or impending emergency. An aging dog is not able to handle disease processes as well as a younger dog; therefore, any illness may lead to more serious complications. If you observe any of the emergency signs, contact your veterinarian as soon as possible. The signs listed below should be considered especially urgent if the problem does not improve or if it worsens. Any changes from the norm for your dog should be considered significant; therefore, if a particular sign is not listed in this section, it should still be considered an important change.

Signs of an Emergency (in addition to the top ten warning signs and the ten signs of cancer)

1. Labored breathing (shallow, rapid or deep)
2. Prolonged or recurring weakness
3. Loss of appetite without return by next meal
4. Bleeding that will not stop
5. Bruising
6. Red or dark spots on the gums
7. Pale or white gums
8. Blue or purple tongue or gums
9. Collapse
10. Cough with difficulty catching breath
11. Bloody or tarry stools
12. Persistent diarrhea
13. Persistent vomiting
14. Vomit that looks like coffee grounds
15. Drooling that will not stop
16. Persistent tearing or rubbing of eye(s)
17. Head tilt

18. Lameness, limping or non-weight bearing on a leg
19. Loss of balance
20. Straining while trying to urinate or defecate
21. Seizures or muscle tremors
22. Dragging toes or leg(s)
23. Paralysis
24. Persistent or recurring pain
25. Distended abdomen
26. Protrusion of any body part
27. Increased or decreased body temperature
28. Unsuccessful attempts at belching or vomiting
29. Inability to climb stairs
30. Crying
31. Pus or unusual discharge from anywhere
32. Sores that do not heal
33. Weight loss
34. Bleeding or discharge from any orifice
35. Offensive odor
36. Difficulty eating or swallowing
37. Weakness, loss of stamina, or hesitation to exercise
38. Increased thirst
39. Broken house habits
40. Weight gain
41. Lumps and Bumps
42. Bad breath
43. Confusion

HEALTH CHECKLIST

Using this health checklist will aid in early detection of disease. Discovering health problems is made easier by knowing what to look for and how to look for it. By becoming familiar with what is normal and what is abnormal, you will be able to understand your dog's symptoms better, and you will be better able to provide information about your dog to your veterinarian. This health checklist will help you identify difficulties early. You should review this list at least twice a month as your dog gets older. If you answer "yes" to any of the following questions, you should contact your veterinarian.

A. **Eyes, Ears, Nose and Throat Checklist**

____ Are the eyes cloudy? Red?

____ Is there discharge coming from the eyes?

____ Is the dog rubbing its eye(s)?

____ Are there any bumps on the dog's eyelids?

____ Is one eye bigger than the other?

____ Is one pupil bigger than the other?

____ Are the eyes moving back and forth when the dog is at rest?

____ Are both eyes affected?

____ Is the head tilted?

____ Is there any discharge coming from the ears?

____ Are the ear flaps swollen?

____ Is there discharge coming from the nose?

    ____ If there is nasal discharge, is it from both nostrils?

    ____ If there is nasal discharge, is it bloody, clear, or cloudy?

____ Are the gums any color other than pink? If so, what color are they? Blue? White?

___ Are there diseased teeth in the mouth?

___ Does the breath smell bad?

___ Is the dog pawing at its mouth?

___ Is the dog drooling?

___ Is there blood in the dog's mouth?

B. Heart and Lungs (Cardiopulmonary) Checklist

___ Is the dog coughing? Is the cough dry or productive (i.e., producing mucus)?

___ Is the dog having difficulty breathing? Does the dog's abdomen move and heave when the pet breathes?

___ Does the dog's abdomen appear enlarged?

___ Has the dog fainted or collapsed?

___ Is the dog wheezing?

    ___ How long have the symptoms been present?

    ___ How long do these spells last?

C. Digestive Tract Checklist

___ Has the dog been vomiting?

    ___ If so, does the food look digested?

    ___ Does the vomit appear as if it has coffee grounds in it?

___ Has the dog missed a meal? How long has it been since the last meal?

___ Has the dog's appetite changed? Has it increased or has it decreased?

___ Is the dog eating only favorite foods?

___ Are the bowel movements abnormal? Soft? Watery? Dry?

___ Is there mucus or blood present in the dog's stool?

___ Are the dog's stools black or clay colored?

___ Is the dog constipated? How long has it been since the last bowel movement?

D. Urinary and Reproductive Tract Checklist

____ Is the dog urinating more frequently?

____ Is the dog urinating less frequently?

____ Is the dog straining to urinate?

____ Is the dog urinating inside the house?

____ Does the dog cry when trying to urinate?

____ Is the dog urinating more volume than usual?

____ Is the dog urinating less volume than usual?

____ Is the dog drinking more water than usual?

____ Is the dog persistently licking its genital area?

____ Is there any discharge coming from the dog's genital area?

E. Integument (Skin) Checklist

____ Are there any hairless areas on the dog?

____ If there are any hairless areas on the dog, are these areas irritated?

____ Is the dog scratching continually?

____ Are there any lumps on the skin? If so, what size?

____ Are there any punctures or lacerations?

____ Is there any evidence of fleas or other external parasites?

____ Is there any evidence of a rash anywhere on the dog's body? If so, where is the rash?

____ Is the skin changing in color and/or texture?

F. Musculoskeletal (Muscle and Bone) & Nervous System Checklist

____ Is the dog unable to move?

____ Is the dog limping? If so, which leg?

____ Is the dog stumbling?

____ Is the dog dragging its legs?

____ Is the dog mentally alert?

____ Does the dog walk in circles?

___ Is the dog uncoordinated?

___ Is the dog having difficulty getting up or down?

___ Does the stiffness get better after the dog is up and moving?

ROUTINE PREVENTIVE HEALTH CARE (ALL AGES)

The best way to prevent problems associated with aging is to maintain proper health care for your pet. Good basic health care is paramount in disease prevention, especially in aging dogs because often they are more susceptible to disease. The old saying "an ounce of prevention is worth a pound of cure" definitely applies to dogs. Many fatal infections can be prevented by proper health care in the form of vaccinations, dental care, spaying/neutering, and regular worm examinations. In fact, proper health care and proper dental care are two simple ways to help your dog live longer and happier.

You have probably heard that for a dog, one year of the pet's life is roughly equivalent to seven years in the life of a person. That means that if your dog gets a physical examination by a veterinarian only once per year, that is equivalent to your getting examined by a doctor only once every seven years. As a dog gets older, the need for medical attention increases, and one year is too long to wait between examinations. Dogs of any age should have a physical examination, performed by a veterinarian, at least every six months. Older dogs, depending upon the breed and the dog's condition, may need even more frequent examinations. Because the life span of a dog is a fraction of the average human life span, six months for a dog represents a substantial period of time.

I. **Infections that Vaccinations Prevent**

A. Distemper – a disease, caused by a virus, that may result in fever, severe respiratory disease and digestive upsets. Usually fatal, this disease may result in permanent neurological problems for dogs that survive.

B. Adenovirus – a disease that may cause respiratory problems or hepatitis (inflammation of the liver).

C. Parainfluenza – a virus that causes respiratory problems.

D. Leptospirosis – a bacterial infection which may result in internal bleeding, digestive upsets, fever and kidney damage.

E. Parvovirus – a highly infectious digestive infection that causes vomiting and severe bloody diarrhea. If not treated, it is usually fatal, with death occurring as soon as 24 hours after the onset of symptoms.

F. Coronavirus – a disease similar to parvovirus except that it is typically not as severe.

G. Bordetella (kennel cough) – a bacterial infection which causes bronchitis resulting in a debilitating cough.

H. Lyme disease – spread by ticks, this disease causes symptoms ranging from depression and loss of appetite to fever, lameness and swollen lymph nodes.

I. Rabies – a disease, transmitted by other infected animals, that is fatal to animals and people.

II. Heartworm Disease

A. Heartworm disease is a contagious parasite (worm) that is spread by mosquitoes. A mosquito bites a dog and deposits, under the skin, larvae which migrate to the heart. Once they are in the heart, the larvae mature into long spaghetti-like worms that interfere with the heart and also cause lung problems.

B. There is no vaccine for heartworm, but there is preventive medication. All dogs that live in heartworm areas should be tested annually and given preventive medication.

III. Dental Care

A. Your dog's teeth should be checked as part of a regular physical examination by your veterinarian.

B. Your veterinarian should recommend food that is appropriate for your dog's dental condition.

C. Foul-smelling breath, loss of appetite and difficulty chewing are all signs of dental problems. If you observe any of these signs, contact your veterinarian.

D. Decayed teeth should either be repaired or removed. Teeth that are decaying and are not treated can result in a serious infection, in addition to causing severe discomfort for your pet.

IV. Elective Surgery – Spaying/Neutering

A. For male dogs, neutering prevents testicular cancer and helps prevent prostatic enlargement and cancer.

B. In female dogs, spaying decreases the risk of uterine cancer and breast cancer.

C. Other benefits of spaying/neutering include:

(1) Prevention of unwanted pregnancies.

(2) Decreased roaming and running away.

(3) For male dogs, improves temperament toward other male dogs and stops marking of territory with urine.

V. Adult Vaccinations and Care

A. Adults not vaccinated as puppies need two vaccinations for all diseases with 3 weeks between shots, except for rabies. Rabies vaccination requires only one starting vaccine with routine booster shots every year to every 3 years.

B. Adults vaccinated as puppies need vaccination boosters every year. Rabies vaccinations may be good for 3 years depending on the type. Check with your dog's veterinarian.

C. Twice per year a veterinarian should check a stool specimen under the microscope for worm eggs or other parasites.

D. Every dog that lives in a heartworm region should be given a blood test once per year to check for the disease, regardless of whether the dog has been taking heartworm preventive medicine all year. The test is necessary because the medicine is not always 100% effective.

E. All dogs in heartworm regions should take heartworm preventive tablets or injections. A single bite from an infected mosquito can transmit the disease.

F. Your dog should have a complete physical examination at least twice each year.

G. Other tests are recommended for aging pets. See pages 40-42.

HEALTH-CARE PROGRAMS

Your veterinarian can work with you and your dog to design a health care plan to suit the needs of your dog. Each plan should be tailored to meet not only the dog's needs but also your budget. Regardless of how you tailor your plan, it should include a minimum of two examinations by a veterinarian each year. These examinations should include a variety of diagnostic tests available to uncover early aging changes in your dog. The examinations and associated tests provide a baseline for comparing future changes, plus they provide valuable information about your dog's internal functions.

I. Tests Available for Aging Dogs

A. Urinalysis – This is a broad range of tests that is conducted on a urine specimen. It provides a great deal of information on everything from kidney and liver functions to diabetes and hormonal diseases, as well as urinary tract infections.

B. Fecal examination – This test is important in detecting parasites that may compromise your dog's health. The fecal specimen is examined with a microscope to check for parasites that frequently cannot be seen by the naked eye. The examination also identifies any blood or mucus, which may be indicative of a variety of ailments.

C. Blood profile – The blood profile is a test that will typically include anywhere from five to fifteen different analyses. It is one of the best tests to screen for changes occurring in the different organs. The blood profile requires only a small amount of blood (an amount equivalent to one teaspoon), yet it can uncover changes in the liver, kidneys, bones, pancreas and much more. It measures the amounts of electrolytes, such as sodium, potassium and phosphorus, which may change in some disease conditions. And typically it includes an analysis of protein levels, which can indicate the presence of certain cancers or other metabolic problems. The test also includes an analysis of your dog's blood sugar level to check for diabetes, a disease that becomes more prevalent as a dog ages.

D.   Complete blood count (CBC) – The CBC is another blood test commonly used to screen for disease. The cost of the test is usually less than that of a blood profile but gives information about the presence of infection, inflammation, blood cancers, anemias, and dehydration by examining the red blood cells and white blood cells. It also checks the platelet count, which is important in clotting. It is important to note that the information that is obtained from this test is quite different from that of the blood profile; one cannot be used to replace the other.

E.   Thyroid analysis – The thyroid analysis is another useful blood test. It is typically performed annually, or any time that a dog shows signs of a thyroid deficiency (such as weight gain, hair loss, lethargy, and/or inability to stay warm).

F.   X-rays (radiographs) – X-rays are performed to screen for aging changes or to further investigate a potential problem. Radiographs are a noninvasive way to look inside a dog to evaluate the size, shape, and position of various organs and to identify the presence of fluids, stones, foreign objects, and/or air in inappropriate places.

G.   Electrocardiogram (ECG or EKG) – The ECG is a noninvasive test that measures electrical changes in the heart. The test can discover arrhythmias (abnormal rhythms of the heart). It can also indirectly confirm heart enlargement and provide information on the seriousness of a heart condition. Some changes in the ECG may also be suggestive of electrolyte imbalances, fluid around the heart, and shock.

H.   Culture – A culture is a test of a sample (e.g., ear discharge, body fluid, or skin) collected from a problem area. With this affordable test, a small specimen is scraped from the area, and the bacteria contained in the specimen are grown in an incubator and then examined for identification. The presence of certain types of bacteria indicates the cause of the problem and enables the veterinarian to treat the condition effectively.

I.   Ultrasound – Ultrasound uses the reflection of sound waves off of internal organs to provide an image of the organs and their surrounding environment. It is similar to an X-ray, except that it uses sound waves, rather than X-rays, to generate the internal picture of the dog's body. Unlike X-rays, it can show pictures of the internal structure of organs, and it can show internal movement, such as the beating of a heart. (An ultrasound of the heart is referred to as a echocardiogram.) Like X-rays, an ultrasound is a noninvasive test.

J.   Endoscopy – With this technique, a fiberoptic scope is used to look inside the body. The scope is passed into the body to examine the surfaces of the digestive tract, respiratory tract or other internal organs. It can be used to retrieve biopsies (samples of tissue) from these areas. It can also be used to retrieve foreign objects from the stomach without using surgery. Anesthesia is usually required.

K.   Biopsies – A biopsy is a tissue sample (i.e., a small piece of skin, bone, muscle, organ or other body cells) which is examined under a microscope to identify abnormalities and thereby make a diagnosis. It is commonly used to determine if a growth is malignant, but it may also diagnose infections and other conditions. The cost of a biopsy is small considering the information it provides and the peace of mind it can provide.

L.   Magnetic Resonance Imaging (MRI) – An MRI is a highly-sophisticated test that uses magnetic waves and computerization to provide a three-dimensional view of areas being examined. It shows contrast of abnormal tissue and can provide some detailed information not available via other diagnostic testing.

M.   Computerized Tomography (CT scan) – a CT scan takes a series of radiographic (X-ray) projections and reorganizes them to create a three-dimensional image that allows for easier recognition of abnormal areas.

II. Geriatric Program First Year

A. Starting age for geriatric program:
   (1) Age 5 for small and medium sized dogs.
   (2) Age 4 to 5 for large dogs.
   (3) Age 4 for giant breeds of dogs.
B. Examination at least once every 6 months.
C. Stool check and urinalysis every 6 months.
D. Heartworm test, complete blood count, and blood profile once per year.
E. Nutrition counseling to determine if diet change is necessary.
F. Other tests, if recommended by your veterinarian, depending upon your dog's health.

III. Geriatric Program Year Two

A. This program builds on the information obtained in the first year of screening.
B. Examination at least once every 6 months.
C. Stool check and urinalysis every 6 months.
D. Heartworm test, complete blood count, profile, and thyroid test at least once per year.
E. Chest X-rays and ECG if a cough, difficult breathing or heart murmur is present.
F. Nutrition counseling to determine if diet change is necessary.
G. Other tests, if recommended by your veterinarian, depending upon the symptoms your dog is exhibiting and the tests results obtained from the above testing.

IV. Geriatric Program Year Three

A. This program builds on the information obtained in the first two years of screening.
B. Examination at least once every 6 months.
C. Stool check and urinalysis every 6 months.
D. Heartworm test every year.
E. Complete blood count, profile, and thyroid test every 6 months if warranted.

F. Nutrition counseling to determine if diet change is necessary.

G. Chest X-rays and ECG as a routine evaluation.

H. Other tests may be recommended by your veterinarian depending upon the symptoms your dog is exhibiting and the tests results.

V. Geriatric Program Year Four

A. This program builds on the information obtained in the first three years of screening.

B. Examination every 4 to 6 months.

C. Stool check and urinalysis every 6 months.

D. Heartworm test once per year.

E. Complete blood count, profile, and thyroid test (every 4 to 6 months or as recommended by your veterinarian).

F. Nutrition counseling to determine if diet change is necessary.

G. Chest X-rays and ECG as a routine evaluation.

H. Other tests should be conducted as recommended by your veterinarian depending upon the symptoms your dog is exhibiting and the tests results obtained from the above testing.

DESIGNING AN EXERCISE PROGRAM

One simple way to help your dog live a longer and happier life is to develop and maintain a proper exercise and weight-control program for your dog. Your dog's exercise program must be tailored to the pet's needs and take into account any health restrictions. Dogs with aging changes must be exercised based on their medical condition. A dog with heart failure may be on a different program from a dog with diabetes. A dog that is overweight but otherwise healthy may require a more rigorous exercise plan than a dog that has kidney failure. Therefore, it is important to consult your veterinarian before starting your dog on any exercise program.

There are general guidelines for exercising dogs. First, start all programs gradually. Start with light exercise on a daily basis. Avoid exercise that is prolonged and not done on a regular schedule, such as going on a weekly hike. Time all daily exercise. If soreness occurs the next day, reduce the intensity and duration of exercise. Ask your veterinarian about pain medicine if soreness develops on a regular basis. Always keep your dog on a leash while exercising near roads.

As an alternative to running or walking, swimming provides good exercise with less wear and tear on the joints. If a dog swims, it must be observed at all times. Dogs can drown while swimming if they fatigue or if a medical problem arises. Life preservers are available for your dog's safety. Make sure that if you are using one of these devices, it is properly balanced for your dog.

Use care when exercising dogs that have poorly developed nostrils (e.g., pugs, bulldogs, Boston terriers, Pekingese, etc.) because they are prone to breathing difficulties and heat stroke. With any dog, on hot days exercise during the coolest part of the day, (i.e., mornings or evenings). Avoid exercising in extremely hot or cold weather. Stop the exercise if your dog shows any discomfort, fatigue, difficulty breathing, or reluctance to continue. If your dog is having difficulty during exercise and is small dog, carry it home. If your dog is difficult to carry, call a friend for a ride home. If a car ride is not available, rest with your dog until all signs disappear. Offer your dog water, if your dog is not vomiting and is alert. Then return home, but divide the walk by resting often before the signs reappear. Contact your veterinarian immediately.

The following suggestions will make exercise for your dog safer and provide a good foundation to build an exercise plan with the assistance of your veterinarian.

I. General Guidelines

A. Consult with your veterinarian before starting any exercise program.

B. Keep your dog on a leash while exercising near roads.

C. Start all programs gradually.

D. On hot days, exercise during the coolest part of the day (i.e., mornings or evenings).

E. Avoid exercising in extremely cold or hot weather.

F. Stop exercise if the dog shows any discomfort, fatigue, difficulty breathing, or reluctance to continue.

G. Take drinking water with you for your dog during exercise sessions.

II. Special Considerations for Dogs with Arthritis

A. Consult with your veterinarian before starting any exercise program.

B. Before any exercise, consider massaging your dog for fifteen minutes to help relieve stiffness. After exercise, another fifteen minutes of massage will help your dog recover better and help prevent soreness.

C. Start with light exercise on a daily basis. Avoid exercise that is prolonged and not done on a regular schedule, such as going on a weekly hike.

D. Consider swimming for your dog as an alternative to running or walking, if the temperature is not too cold. (Water temperature should be at least 65 degrees Fahrenheit.) Swimming provides good exercise with minimal wear and tear on the joints.

E.   Time all daily exercise. If your dog shows signs of being sore the next day, reduce the intensity and/or duration of future exercise.

F.   Plan a complete exercise program that you can adjust to suit your dog's changing needs. For some dogs it is appropriate to increase exercise over time, whereas with others it is necessary to decrease exercise over time. The following is an example of an exercise program for an arthritic dog:

Week One
1.   Ideally, provide 15 minutes of body massage prior to exercise to warm/stretch your dog's muscles.
2.   10 minutes of easy walking twice daily for 1 week.
3.   Ideally, provide 15 minutes of body massage after exercise to warm/stretch your dog's muscles.
4.   If your dog seems to be in pain during exercise or the next day, decrease the exercise to 5 minutes per session.

Week Two
1.   Same as Week One, except increase exercise time by 50% (e.g., from 10 minutes twice per day to 15 minutes twice per day) or add 5 minutes of swimming in calm water that is 65 degrees Fahrenheit or warmer).
2.   If your dog seems to be in pain during exercise or the next day, decrease the exercise time by half (e.g., from 15 minutes to 7 1/2 minutes).

Week Three
1.   Same as Week Two, except either increase the duration of exercise by another 25% to 50% or else add short sessions of jogging to the exercise. When jogging, try 10-15 yard increments combined with walking.
2.   If your dog seems to be in pain during exercise or the next day, decrease the exercise by reducing the time or decreasing the jogging.

III. Special Considerations for Dogs with Medical Conditions

A. Consult with your veterinarian before starting any exercise program.

B. Follow all instructions from General Guidelines above, page 46.

C. Watch for any signs of fatigue during exercise (e.g., difficulty breathing, loss of strength or coordination, confusion, reluctance to continue, etc.). If you observe any signs of fatigue, stop exercising immediately.

D. During exercise, watch for any signs of illness, such as vomiting, diarrhea, confusion, loss of coordination or difficulty breathing.

　　1. If any of these signs are noted, stop all exercise. If your dog is small carry the dog home. If your dog is difficult to carry, call for a car ride home. If a car ride is not available, rest with your dog until all signs disappear; then return home, but divide the walk by resting often before the signs reappear.

　　2. Offer water if your dog is not vomiting and is alert.

　　3. Contact your veterinarian immediately.

PART 3

—

PHYSICAL PROBLEMS

INTRODUCTION TO PROBLEMS

This section is designed to provide a reference for learning about problems that commonly affect older dogs. The topics, listed in alphabetical order, include a variety of conditions, symptoms, diseases and miscellaneous difficulties. If your dog has been diagnosed with a particular condition or disease, then you can look up the information directly by going to that topic. If you and/or your veterinarian observe certain symptoms but a diagnosis has not yet been made, you should look up the symptom(s) that you observe and learn how you might make your dog more comfortable.

Regardless of the problem, there are some basic steps you can take to ensure that your dog's needs are properly met. The following information will enable you to take appropriate action in a variety of situations.

I.   Basic Steps in an Emergency

A.   Focus on the dog's needs, and use common sense. If you are unable to deal with the situation, then delegate the care to someone else.

B.   Seek assistance by calling the dog's veterinarian. If the problem occurs outside of regular veterinary hours, call for after-hour help.

C.   If you suspect poisoning and cannot reach a veterinarian, call your local poison control hotline or the National Animal Poison Control Center. (The ASPCA Animal Poison Control Center provides assistance for a fee – $45 at the time of this printing: 1-800-548-2423.) Do not wait to see if your pet develops symptoms; delay in treating for poisoning may be fatal.

E.   If no professional help is available:
(1) Confine the dog.
(2) Keep the dog quiet and warm.

(3) If you own a copy of the book *Emergency First Aid For Your Dog* by Dr. Tamara Shearer, refer to that book. If not, refer to the Appendix on Basic First Aid.

(4) Note any and all symptoms.

(5) Observe whether the condition is getting better, staying the same or getting worse.

II. Basic Steps in a Nonemergency Situation

A. Contact a veterinarian as soon as possible.

B. Observe all signs of the problem, and note any changes that may occur.

ANAL GLAND/SAC ABSCESS

Aging dogs, especially those that are overweight, are at higher risk of developing problems with their anal glands. Anal glands (also called anal sacs) are located along both sides of the rectum (at the 4 o'clock and 8 o'clock positions). They serve no known useful function for the dog. The glands normally fill with a foul-smelling secretion that is discharged from the glands through small ducts during bowel movements. On occasion, these glands become infected or the ducts become plugged, and the secretion builds. Dogs experiencing discomfort with their anal glands may first show signs of scooting their rear ends on the floor or ground. They may also show swelling around the rectum. Other signs include difficulty sitting and persistent licking of the rectum. If the glands become blocked, the pressure in the glands can become so great that the gland and the skin over the area break open, and blood, pus and foul discharge spill out. Anal gland difficulties may occur in any breed of dog but are most common in smaller breeds of dogs.

Anal gland infections are painful, but there is a procedure you can use to help treat the condition and lessen the pain. As with any situation where your dog is in pain, you may need to use a muzzle to ensure that your pet does not bite as a reaction to your handling. However, use a muzzle only if the dog is not having difficulty breathing and has not been vomiting. If at any time the dog has difficulty breathing, remove the muzzle. Also, do not use a muzzle if your dog has a flat face (e.g., a pug, boxer, English bulldog, etc.).

To treat infected anal glands, fill a bathtub with warm water, and have the dog sit in the tub for 10 to 20 minutes. If the dog is not in too much pain, cleanse the area under its tail with shampoo and then rinse well. Dry the dog with a towel. Apply antibiotic ointment (e.g., Polysporin®) to any open wounds. If necessary, apply an Elizabethan collar to prevent the dog from licking its rectum. (An Elizabethan collar is a cone-shaped device that fits around the dog's neck and prevents the dog from being able to lick itself. See pages 239-240.) Contact a veterinarian for additional care. A veterinarian may need to further cleanse and flush the abscess and open up the ducts leading from the gland. Also, your veterinarian may need to prescribe pain medication and antibiotics to combat the infection.

How to Treat Condition and Improve Comfort

A. You may wish to use a muzzle to prevent being bitten when you treat your dog. However, use a muzzle only if the dog is not having difficulty breathing and has not been vomiting. If at any time the dog has difficulty breathing, remove the muzzle. Also, do not use a muzzle if your dog has a flat face (e.g., a pug, boxer, English bulldog, etc.).

B. Fill a bathtub with warm water, and have the dog sit in the tub for 10 to 20 minutes.

C. If the dog is not in too much pain, cleanse the area under its tail with shampoo, and then rinse well. Dry the dog with a towel.

D. Apply antibiotic ointment (e.g., Polysporin®) to any open wounds.

E. If necessary, apply an Elizabethan collar to prevent the dog from licking its rectum.

F. Contact a veterinarian for additional care.

ANEMIA

Anemia is a condition characterized by insufficient red cells in the blood resulting in an inability of the blood to carry an adequate amount of oxygen for normal physical needs. In dogs there are many causes, but, unlike in humans, iron deficiency is rarely one of them. The effects of anemia on aging dogs can be very debilitating and can make affected dogs more susceptible to other health problems.

The signs of anemia include listlessness or depression, pale or white gums, loss of appetite, labored breathing, and/or collapse. Diagnosis of anemia is usually made through blood tests. Determining the cause of anemia sometimes requires further testing, such as a bone marrow biopsy.

There are two general causes of anemia: (1) loss of blood, and (2) an inability of the body to produce or maintain enough red blood cells. Blood loss from trauma is the most common cause of anemia in dogs, but anemia from blood loss can also occur when there is internal bleeding unrelated to trauma (e.g., from cancers and ulcers, which are conditions common in older dogs). Also fleas and parasites can sometimes consume enough blood to cause anemia.

Red blood cells are manufactured in the bone marrow, and certain conditions affect the bone marrow's ability to produce blood cells. Cancers, drugs, and chronic kidney failure can affect the bone marrow, as can poisonings, chronic or long-term diseases and nutritional deficiencies. Another common cause of anemia in older dogs is a condition called immune-mediated hemolytic anemia, a condition in which the dog's immune system attacks its own red blood cells. This condition most often affects female dogs. It is important that a veterinarian determines the cause of the anemia so that appropriate treatment can be administered.

Treatment may range from giving antibiotics and immune suppressant drugs to giving a transfusion and anabolic steroids. The outcome of the disease is dependent upon the cause and proper treatment.

I. Signs of Anemia (some or all may be present)

A. Listlessness

B. Depression

C. Pale or white gums

D. Loss of appetite

E. Labored breathing

F. Collapse

II. Immediate Action for Dogs with Suspected Anemia

A. Contact your veterinarian. Early diagnosis and treatment may be critical to the outcome. Your veterinarian can perform tests to determine the cause of the anemia and its seriousness.

B. If your dog is having difficulty breathing, avoid all stress. The least bit of stress may precipitate a crisis when the pet cannot breathe. Plan the handling of the dog to minimize excitement. Never hold the dog tightly. Never lay the dog on its back or side because this will compromise oxygen exchange by putting extra pressure on the chest.

III. Additional Precautions for Dogs with Suspected Anemia

A. Make sure the dog's diet is properly balanced and formulated. Do not feed your dog table scraps as a replacement for commercial dog food.

B. Ask your veterinarian about vitamins. Vitamin supplements may help prevent further complications of the anemia.

C. Decrease the amount of exercise according to the severity of the condition.

D. Carefully follow your veterinarian's instructions for medications and rechecks.

ARTHRITIS (OSTEOARTHRITIS/ DEGENERATIVE JOINT DISEASE)

Osteoarthritis or degenerative joint disease is common in the aging dog. In fact, it is probably the leading cause of disability in dogs. Osteoarthritis occurs when the cartilage lining the joint surface breaks down and bone is deposited in the joint. As a joint ages, the cartilage lining the joint changes in its chemical makeup and becomes more easily damaged. The degenerative joint disease in dogs usually occurs from three sources: (1) normal aging changes of the joint surfaces, (2) damage to the joint from a previous injury, and/or (3) developmental problems such as hip dysplasia (poorly developed hip joint) or patellar luxations (slipping of the knee cap).

The signs of osteoarthritis include stiffness (especially after resting for long periods or after extended exercise), reluctance to rise, hesitation in climbing or jumping, and crying when moving. Physical changes include loss of muscle tone, loss of muscle mass of affected area, swelling over the affected joint and/or pain over the affected joint. Diagnosis is usually through a thorough physical examination and X-rays.

The area of the dog's body most commonly affected by degenerative joint disease is the hind end. When the hind end is affected, the dog experiences difficulty rising from a sitting or lying position.

Degenerative joint disease along the spine is referred to as spondylosis. Spondylosis is common in older dogs, especially older large breeds, and is particularly common in boxers, Labradors and German shepherds. With spondylosis, bone spurs develop on the vertebrae, sometimes fusing the spine together. The bony growth may compress nerves, making it hard for the dog to get up. Some dogs will walk with an exaggerated arched or straight back.

Providing a proper exercise and weight-control program for your dog is the most important measure you can take to help prevent arthritis or to keep an arthritic dog comfortable. Depending upon your dog's condition, certain types of exercise may minimize wear and tear on arthritic joints while still providing good exercise (e.g., swimming). Diet is important because an overweight dog will have more difficulty supporting its weight on sore joints compared to a fit dog. Consult your veterinarian to determine the amount and type of exercise and type of diet that is best suited for your dog.

A dog with osteoarthritis should require strict rest only if there is a sudden painful spell. Most commonly, pain control is managed with anti-inflammatory drugs. The newer anti-inflammatory drugs are more effective with fewer side effects than the older preparations. However, drug therapy is secondary to weight control and exercise. Nutritional supplements, such as glucosamine and chondroitin sulfate, and certain fish oils, might also be of benefit. In addition, acupuncture and massage can often provide significant relief. Ask your veterinarian.

Never give any medications to your dog without first consulting your veterinarian. Unprescribed medicines may be harmful to your dog, plus they may mask symptoms the veterinarian will need to see in order to make a proper diagnosis and prescribe proper treatment.

WARNING: Tylenol® (acetaminophen) and Advil®/Motrin® (ibuprofen) are toxic to dogs. Tylenol® cannot be metabolized by the liver and may result in liver failure. Liver failure may be preceded by loss of appetite, weakness, blue gums, difficult breathing, vomiting, diarrhea, and/or the presence of dark urine. Ibuprofen causes severe stomach ulcers and sometimes liver and kidney disease; symptoms include vomiting, diarrhea, listlessness, increased thirst, and/or increased urinations.

There are many things you can do to keep an arthritic dog comfortable. Providing appropriate bedding is important. Good bedding will insulate the dog from cold floors and thereby help prevent stiffness commonly caused by lying on a cold hard surface. Because it is important that the bedding you use is kept clean, you should select bedding material that is easy to wash. The size of the bed should be big enough to allow the dog to stretch out and lie flat. Its thickness depends on the type of material used, but should be thick enough to provide insulation from the floor and provide soft padding. Soft padding is important to prevent bed sores from developing. Examples of appropriate bedding include folded comforters, commercial stuffed beds with a removable, waterproof cover, and rubber mats covered with a blanket or towels. Materials such as foam should be avoided unless a waterproof covering is available.

57

Waterbeds, even though easy to clean, need to be large enough for comfort and carefully monitored for proper temperature.

A dog's bed should be situated in a draft free, dry, well ventilated area. This area should be in a well-supervised part of the house so that you can interact with the dog and thereby observe the dog's habits. Try to avoid dark, damp basements as well as the cold outdoors. Make sure that the dog's food and water are near the bed to provide easy access for the dog.

Some owners like to have their dog sleep in bed with them. If you are one of these owners but your dog has difficulty getting into the bed because of arthritis, you might consider putting a stepping stool beside the bed. While smaller dogs may be lifted onto or off of a bed, by creating a means for the dog to come and go under its own power, the dog will have greater access to food and water and toys or anything else. If your dog is too debilitated to make use of a stepping stool, you may wish to consider building a plywood ramp; but make sure the ramp is at a low angle, and make sure it has a rail on both sides that the dog can balance against.

Dogs with osteoarthritis have difficulty getting up from a seated or lying position. Although smaller dogs might be lifted and carried without effort, it is important to help a dog of any size to stand. Helping the dog to stand, rather than carrying it, will help preserve the dog's muscle strength, improve its circulation, and provide ample opportunity for the dog to go to the bathroom.

Note that proper footing is essential for enabling an arthritic dog to get up and move about. Slippery floors are hazardous for older dogs and should be covered with nonskid throw rugs, bath mats or industrial rubber mats. Towels and blankets are not recommended as floor coverings because they are too slippery.

If your dog has good front leg strength but has difficulty rising from a sitting or lying position because of problems with its hind quarters, there is a technique you can use to help. Place a towel under the dog's abdomen (as illustrated on page 161), and use the towel as a sling to help lift the dog. To help a dog that has weakness in both front and rear legs, use one towel as a sling between the front legs and another towel under the dog's abdomen as a sling for the rear legs. Lift the front towel first, and once the front end is almost up, start to lift the back towel. You may, if you have one available, substitute a log carrier for the towels. Note that whenever you are assisting a dog in rising from a seated or lying position, the dog is depending upon you for its balance; make sure the dog does not stumble and hit its nose on the ground.

58

A dog with front end difficulties only can be helped up by running a towel between the front legs and then lifting using the towel as a sling. This method may be facilitated by grasping and gently pulling up on the collar at the same time. See the illustrations on page 163.

Going from a standing position to a sitting or lying position may also be a problem for an arthritic dog. You may help by tucking the back legs under the dog if you see the dog struggling to sit or lie down. You may also be of assistance simply by providing a support for the dog to brace itself against as it attempts to bend its legs, and the support might be nothing more than your own legs as you stand beside the dog. You might also try placing large, soft pillows around the dog to allow for a graduated transition from the up to the down position, but make sure the pillows are not slippery against the floor.

Some dogs with advanced arthritis are unable to stand or move without your complete support. To lift and move a medium sized to large dog that does not have the strength to get up on its own, put one arm under the dog's stomach (below the ribs) and the other hand under the dog's neck (with the dog's neck in the corner formed by your elbow). When lifting the dog, bend your knees and lift with equal pressure on both arms. If your strength does not permit you to lift the dog, tuck a blanket under the dog or roll the dog onto a blanket and pull the dog on the blanket or have someone lift opposite corners.

Contact your veterinarian if there is any change in your dog's ability to get up and down. Also, contact your veterinarian if you are unable to move your dog.

Arthritis Checklist

A. If you suspect that your dog may be developing arthritis, contact your veterinarian. One or more signs may be present, including:
   1. Stiffness after periods of resting
   2. Stiffness after extended exercise
   3. Reluctance to rise
   4. Hesitation in climbing or jumping
   5. Crying when moving
   6. Loss of muscle tone or muscle mass
   7. Swelling and/or pain over affected joint

B. If the dog is overweight, start a weight reduction plan approved by your veterinarian. Your doctor may recommend foods that are low in Calories and high in fiber.

C. Ask your veterinarian about an appropriate exercise plan to help keep your dog's muscles toned. See pages 45-48.

D. Do not restrict activity except or unless the dog experiences a sudden painful event.

E. Contact your veterinarian regarding supplements that may help decrease damage to the cartilage.

F. Ask your veterinarian about medicines to help control pain. Never give your dog human medications without the advice of a veterinarian. Note that Tylenol® (acetaminophen) and Advil®/Motrin® (ibuprofen) are toxic to dogs.

G. Provide proper bedding
   1. Make sure the bed is large enough for the dog to lie flat.
   2. Make sure the bed is clean and dry. Do not use foam for bedding unless it has a waterproof covering.
   3. Locate the bed in a draft-free, dry, well-ventilated environment where the dog can be closely monitored.

H. Keep food and water in close proximity to ensure that your dog's arthritis does not prevent proper hydration and nourishment.

I. If necessary, assist your dog in rising from a sitting or lying position as illustrated on pages 161 and 163.

BEHAVIOR CHANGES

One of the more frustrating challenges for any owner of an older dog is coping with the behavioral changes that the dog will tend to undergo. These changes may appear suddenly, or they may start gradually but eventually reach a point where they are difficult for an owner to endure. Behavioral problems that older dogs commonly encounter include broken house-training habits, separation anxiety, increased vocalization, destructive behaviors and problems resulting from senility. Because many behavioral problems have a medical origin, treatment of any disruptive behavior should be directed at the cause of the problem rather than directed at the behavior itself. Punishment is counterproductive because it serves only to frighten the dog and does nothing for the underlying difficulty. You should discuss any behavioral change with your veterinarian, even changes not specifically mentioned above.

A dog's past behavioral history will influence its behavior throughout the aging process. As a dog ages, personality traits tend to become more pronounced. A dog that is timid as a puppy will likely become even more timid as an adult, whereas an aggressive puppy will tend to become more combative with age, unless behavioral modification is initiated. In addition to a dog's past, another factor that contributes to the dog's behavior, or changes in behavior, is the loss or decline of sight, hearing, and/or smell. A decline in these senses may exacerbate existing tendencies and cause more pronounced behavioral characteristics; a dog may become more timid or more aggressive or more destructive. Also, aging dogs are more sensitive than younger dogs to events that can change behavior.

Broken House Habits – Compared with younger dogs, older dogs have a higher incidence of losing their housebreaking habits. This change is often medical rather than behavioral in its origin. Many disease conditions may cause your dog to lose control of urination and bowel movements. Urinary incontinence can be caused by bladder irritations, decreased levels of the hormone estrogen, excess cortisol hormone, nerve degeneration, and various aging changes of internal organs. Loss of control of bowel movements may be caused by any condition causing irritation of the bowels, including

61

dietary indiscretions, intestinal parasites, changes of internal organ function, inflammation, nerve degeneration, and certain cancers. Physical causes must be investigated before concluding that a dog is experiencing a purely behavioral problem. Because the volume and frequency of accidents may be helpful in determining whether a problem is medical or behavioral, you should note this information and provide it to your dog's veterinarian.

Treatment of your dog to get rid of the problem of house soiling is a three-fold process. First, you must eliminate any medical complications or conditions that may be contributing to the problem. This could include treating for direct causes, such as a bladder infection, parasites or hormonal changes, or indirect causes resulting from conditions that impede the pet's mobility (e.g., arthritis or obesity). Second, you must make sure that the house soiling is not a reaction to an event or circumstance (e.g., separation anxiety or other stress reaction as discussed on pages 24-26). If the cause is an event or circumstance, you must identify and then eliminate it. Then third, after items 1 and 2 above have been ruled out or else adequately addressed, you must retrain the dog to establish the proper habits again. For retraining, start by taking the dog outside to go to the bathroom every 2-4 hours. Also, if the dog has difficulty with mobility (e.g., if the dog suffers from arthritis) assist it in getting up and going outside. Refer to the chapter on arthritis, pages 56-60, for methods to improve and assist your dog's mobility.

Paper training or diapering may be a solution for an older dog. Modifying feeding times and, in certain circumstances, changing food type may decrease the volume of stool produced. Restricting water intake is generally inadvisable and should be done only under the specific advice of your dog's veterinarian. It is important to note that restricting water with certain disease conditions and medications can be life threatening.

Remember, never punish a dog for having accidents in the house; save your effort to modify the problem that causes the accident.

Separation Anxiety and Destructive Behavior – Older dogs frequently suffer from a condition called separation anxiety. Separation anxiety is characterized by disruptive and/or destructive behaviors that occur shortly after the owner leaves the home. These behaviors may include excessive vocalization (e.g., howling, barking and whining), urinating or defecating in the house, chewing, and digging. Dogs suffering from separation anxiety may also exhibit loss of appetite and depression whenever the owner is away. Medical problems may develop, such as vomiting and diarrhea. When the owner returns, the dog may show uncontrollable excitability.

Dogs develop separation anxiety for a variety of reasons. Separation anxiety is not a result of lack of training but rather a response to stress. Abandonment is frequently a key issue; either the dog perceives itself at risk for abandonment resulting from some present circumstances, or the dog reacts to having been abandoned previously, or the dog develops strong bonds to a person and the absence of that person makes the dog feel abandoned. Examples of experiences of a dog that may lead to separation anxiety include being left alone in a strange place, being boarded at a kennel for an extended period of time, and extended vacations or business trips by the primary owner. In addition, specific events that frighten the dog, even common events such as thunderstorms, can cause the dog to become afraid to be alone and lead to separation anxiety. Older dogs in particular are more sensitive to traumatic events.

Treatment of separation anxiety and its accompanying disruptive or destructive behavior should be directed at the cause of the problem. Punishment is counterproductive because it serves only to frighten the dog and does nothing for the underlying difficulty. Crate training does little to correct separation anxiety. It will protect the surrounding environment, but it will not help the dog's anxiety. To treat separation anxiety, practice short departures from the home. You should attempt to return from the departures before the dog exhibits any bad behaviors. Try leaving on a television or radio for background noise. Desensitize your dog to anxiety triggers; for example,, if picking up your keys is an anxiety trigger, then perhaps you should try picking up your keys often without leaving. A special toy may also be presented to the dog as a safety cue that lets the dog know you will be back. In order to be effective, this safety-cue technique requires that you make an expedient return before the dog reacts to its anxiety. Otherwise the dog will not form an association between the toy and your safe return. Another technique that may help your dog grow more accustomed to being left alone is to make the dog stay alone in a separate room at times while you are at home. Also, you may try restricting the dog from sleeping with you in your bedroom or even restricting lap sitting. Antianxiety drugs often complement training of the dog. Also, videotaping your dog's behavior when you are away may provide insights into the dog's problem.

One method of assessing the progress of your dog's

separation anxiety is to note the apparent level of anxiety at the time of departure and the level of excitement upon your return; if your dog is improving, both the anxiety and the excitement will tend to decrease.

Increased Vocalization – It is not normal for a healthy dog to suddenly develop a problem with excessive barking. Barking is the dog's way of communicating, and although it may simply seem like a nuisance noise, there is always a reason for every type of behavior.

Treatment of any disruptive behavior should be directed at the cause of the problem. Punishment is counterproductive because it serves only to frighten the dog and does nothing for the underlying difficulty. Rather than punish a dog for barking, try to determine if the barking is a response to a medical problem, separation anxiety, hunger or noise or anything else. Then, work to eliminate the cause. If you are unable to identify the cause, ask your veterinarian.

If you have a breed that tends to be particularly vocal, or if your particular dog simply happens to be especially vocal, there are some solutions to the barking. In particular, there are special collars that have been developed to provide negative reinforcement for barking. Some emit a citronella spray, and others emit a high-pitched tone. The spray collars are safe and usually effective. Avoid shock collars. Ask your veterinarian which collar might be appropriate for your dog.

Senility – Senile degeneration is a disorder in which the dog undergoes a decline in mental activity that leads to dullness, decreased response, increased sleep time, confusion and forgetfulness. The dog may lose interest in food, people and other animals. It may stop responding to commands and may lose its house-training habits. While there are diseases and medical conditions that can cause these symptoms, senile degeneration can occur in an aging dog without the presence of any other problems and without any identifiable origin. Medical conditions causing signs of senile degeneration (such as organ failure, diabetes, cancers, etc.) must be eliminated before a diagnosis of senility can be made. Consult your veterinarian regarding medications to help lessen the symptoms of senility.

The following guidelines summarize help for certain behavioral problems.

How to Respond to Behavioral Changes

A. Report any behavioral change to your veterinarian.

B. Always consider the possibility that there is a medical cause to the behavioral problem.

C. Never punish your dog for barking, being anxious, being confused or house soiling. Instead, investigate and eliminate the underlying cause of the problem.

D. Correct the problem as soon as it is recognized.

E. For house breaking accidents, the dog may need to be retrained.

   1. Take the dog outside every 2-4 hours.

   2. Make it easy for the dog to get outside. Provide good footing and/or build a ramp.

   3. Modify feeding times.

   4. Consider paper training or, if severe, diapering.

F. For separation anxiety, attempt to reduce the dog's anxiety.

   1. Provide background noise when you are away (e.g., turn on a radio or television when you leave the dog).

   2. Take only short trips away from the dog.

   3. Give the dog a special toy each time you leave.

   4. Make sure the dog is not disruptive because it is hungry, cold or sick.

BLINDNESS

Loss of vision in older dogs may result from several causes. The loss of sight is usually gradual in nature, which gives the dog time to adjust to the change. There are numerous early signs of vision loss in an aging dog. The dog may start bumping into things, especially at night or in dark rooms, or the dog may become unresponsive to movements in its field of vision. Blindness may be associated with a change in the appearance of the eyes, such as increased size, tearing, or cloudiness. Pain from glaucoma may be exhibited by the dog rubbing its face. A dog's gait may change into a high-stepping, animated one to keep from stumbling. The dogs may also become more sensitive to sound and touch. Sometimes loss of vision may evoke behavior changes. During loss of vision, different sizes, shapes, and motions of objects or people may be confusing; the dog may respond with aggression, confusion, or fear.

Dogs typically adjust well to gradual loss of vision. They are able to rely on their other senses, particularly smell and hearing, to compensate. Even if the sense of hearing is diminished, they still tend to do well, especially in familiar surroundings. In fact, your dog's ability to compensate with other senses may make you unaware of the existence of a vision problem.

The most common causes of blindness in dogs include cataracts, retinal disease, and corneal disease. Cataracts occur in dogs when an opacity (dense spot) develops in the lens and blocks the passage of light. Cataracts usually cause a gradual loss of vision. They can be caused by normal aging changes of the lens or by disease processes that affect the lens. Diseases that promote the development of cataracts include diabetes, malnutrition, and inflammations. A cataract is described by its size, shape, age of onset, and its opacity.

Treatment of cataracts is best accomplished by surgery. The surgery entails the removal and replacement of the lens. Prior to surgery, a test called an electroretinogram is run to make sure that other than cataract difficulty, there is vision in the eye.

There is one condition that a dog owner may mistakenly think is a cataract. Lenticular sclerosis is a condition whereby the lens becomes thickened with age and the eye appears cloudy. This

66

cloudiness does not interfere with vision. The two conditions (cataract versus lenticular sclerosis) can be distinguished through a routine eye examination by a veterinarian.

The retina is the back lining inside the eye which receives the light through the lens and sends signals to the brain for interpretation. There are several conditions that affect the retina in aging dogs. One problem is progressive retinal atrophy (i.e., a gradual degeneration of the retina). This condition commonly affects poodles. The disease process is gradual, starting with loss of vision at night and can eventually lead to total blindness. Unfortunately, at present there is no effective treatment for this condition.

Another retinal condition that can cause blindness is a detached retina. When a detached retina occurs, the retina pulls away from its normal position. This condition may occur suddenly and may result in immediate and total blindness. The cause may be anything from high blood pressure to trauma to diabetes or other diseases. Treatment for a detached retina will depend upon the particular circumstances. Certain medicines may encourage reattachment in some cases. Surgery is less successful with dogs than with people, and corrective surgery for dogs is not widely available. Any treatment for a detached retina will be ineffective unless the underlying cause is first eliminated. In other words, if the cause is high blood pressure, the high blood pressure must be treated.

Aging dogs are also prone to developing diseases that affect the cornea (the transparent covering of the eye). These problems include infections and lack of tear production (keratoconjunctivitis sicca). Cysts or tumors on the eyelids may cause abrasion to the corneas leading to decreased vision. Most eye infections are treated with antibiotics, whereas tear production difficulties are treated with artificial tears and/or medications to stimulate tear production.

Glaucoma can be a problem with aging dogs. Glaucoma is a disease characterized by a build-up of pressure inside the eye to a point where damage may occur to the retina and optic nerve, often resulting in blindness. Although glaucoma is not as common as many other eye problems, it is serious, and it requires prompt treatment to prevent permanent damage. One symptom of glaucoma is pain in the affected eye or eyes. The pain may be evidenced by the dog rubbing and pawing at its face. Also, the cornea may take on a cloudy or white appearance, and the affected eye may appear enlarged and/or the pupil may be dilated. Glaucoma is considered a medical emergency because the build-up of pressure can cause blindness in a short time. Glaucoma is most often diagnosed through a routine eye examination by a veterinarian. It is treated with special oral and eye medicines.

Routine eye examinations at least once every six months by your veterinarian should identify early signs of eye problems and help prevent many serious or permanent vision problems. However, over time your dog's vision will likely deteriorate to some extent simply from the aging process, and it is important to know what to do to make sure your pet is best able to cope with its diminished vision. The following suggestions will help your dog adjust to loss of sight.

Recommended Actions to Help a Dog with Diminished Vision

A. If you suspect that your dog may be losing its sight, contact your veterinarian.

B. Increase verbal commands.

C. Keep the surrounding environment stable or teach the dog where things have moved.

D. Keep rooms well lit.

E. Review yard boundaries.

F. Block off stairs.

G. Avoid confusing or erratic movements.

BREATHING DIFFICULTIES
OR
RESPIRATORY DISTRESS

A dog suffering from breathing difficulties or respiratory distress does not receive enough oxygen to be comfortable or function normally. The condition may be caused by a variety of disease processes, but regardless of the cause, the signs are similar. The dog may take short, shallow, rapid breaths or may pant. Or the dog's breathing may be deeper with a noticeable contraction of the abdominal muscles. The dog's gum or tongue color may be purple, blue, pale pink, or white. The pet may be able only to sit upright with its elbows pointed outward; the dog may not be able to lie flat. The dog may be depressed, but sometimes restless, due to the lack of oxygen. There may be other signs of illness, such as confusion, vomiting, diarrhea, or seizures. When the lack of oxygen is severe, the dog may collapse and stop breathing.

There are many causes of breathing difficulty. They include, but are not limited to, heart disease, lung disease, heat stroke, internal bleeding, shock, trauma, anemia, fractured ribs, poisonings, obstruction of the airway, smoke inhalation, and most other medical emergencies. Regardless of the cause, breathing difficulty is considered a medical emergency. Contact a veterinarian immediately if you observe any of the breathing difficulty signs listed above. Diagnosis of the underlying difficulty is usually made through physical examination, blood tests, and X-rays. Treatment must be directed at the underlying cause of the breathing difficulty.

The following suggestions will help keep the dog comfortable until a veterinarian can be reached.

How to Improve Comfort

A. Avoid all stress. The least amount of stress may precipitate a crisis when your dog cannot breathe properly.

B. Plan the handling of your dog to minimize excitement. Never

69

hold your dog tightly.

C. Keep your dog in an upright position (i.e., belly down). Never lay the dog on its back or side because those positions put extra pressure on the chest and make breathing more difficult.

D. Contact a veterinarian immediately.

CANCERS

As a dog ages, it is at high risk of developing cancers. Cancer (also called "malignancy") refers to a group of abnormal cells that grows quickly, invades, and/or spreads throughout the body. The different types of cancers may affect any area of the body and any organ, including the blood, bones, brain, breasts, skin, pancreas and liver. Certain types of cancers progress slower than others and cause only minimal discomfort in their early stages. Dogs that have these types of cancers may lead a contented lifestyle for some time. Over time, however, a dog with any cancer is likely to develop complications associated with the disease, and these complications may shorten the dog's lifespan. Early detection of cancer helps improve the dog's chances of recovery, plus it provides you with the knowledge necessary to ensure that your pet is as comfortable as possible for as long as possible. Common signs of cancer in animals include:

1. Any sore that will not heal
2. Bleeding or discharge from any body opening
3. Abnormal lumps, bumps, growths or swellings that persist, regardless of whether they continue to grow
4. Loss of appetite or difficulty eating or swallowing
5. Weight loss (may or may not be accompanied by loss of appetite)
6. Offensive odor in general or from a particular area
7. Difficulty breathing, loss of energy, weakness or lack of stamina
8. Persistent limping, lameness or stiffness
9. Difficulty urinating or defecating, or increased time required to urinate or defecate
10. A general decline in health, or behavior that seems to indicate rapid aging

If you observe any of the above warning signs, contact your veterinarian. If your dog does have cancer, proper diagnosis may enable effective treatment, which might include surgery, radiation therapy, chemotherapy, holistic medicine, or treatment of cancer side effects. The type of treatment depends on the specific cancer as well

71

as the progression of the disease. Depending upon the type and severity of the cancer, the goal of treatment may be to cure the disease, to accomplish remission, or to lessen the symptoms of the cancer and thereby improve the dog's comfort.

Tending to any complications from the cancer may enable your pet to be comfortable and enjoy a longer life. For example, if your dog suffers from weight loss or a decrease in appetite from the disease, your pet's diet can be adjusted by your veterinarian to provide more nutrition in smaller quantities.

How to Improve Comfort for a Dog that has Cancer

A. Report any changes in behavior or health to your veterinarian.

B. Frequent veterinary examinations may be necessary to determine the need to change any treatment to prolong your dog's life and provide comfort.

C. Medications can be used to prevent further deterioration or lessen complications.

D. Fresh water should always be available. Never withhold water from an older dog unless the dog is vomiting or unless you are advised to do so by your veterinarian.

E. Increase access to water by placing several water bowls throughout the house, including where the dog lies.

F. Make sure your dog gets proper nourishment
   1. Nutritional consultation and diet change may be recommended according to your dog's age, weight, medical status, and veterinarian's recommendation.
   2. Make sure your dog's food is fresh.
   3. Feed your dog food that is recommended by your veterinarian. Human food should be used only as a last resort if your dog refuses to eat recommended dog food.
   4. A different diet may increase interest in food, but make sure any dietary changes are made gradually and follow your veterinarian's recommendations.
   5. If your dog is reluctant to eat, try warming the food, or try adding water, bouillon, clam juice, or garlic to enhance the food.
   6. Serving food in the presence of other animals may increase

72

your dog's appetite.

7. Human companionship through hand feeding, petting and talking may encourage your dog to eat.

8. Feed your dog several small meals throughout the day.

G. Avoid stressing pets that have cancer or any chronic disease.

H. Help your dog go outside to go the bathroom at least four times per day.

I. Keep your dog clean and dry.

CHRONIC ILLNESSES

Chronic illnesses are diseases with a long duration or diseases with frequent reoccurrences. Unlike acute problems, which occur suddenly giving pets little time to adjust to disease changes, chronic diseases occur gradually, enabling your dog to adjust to changes in body function without suffering many side effects. However, over time, chronic illnesses eventually tend to result in the loss of one or more organ functions and lead to a decline in your dog's condition.

Regardless of the type of chronic illness, there are some common symptoms. As a chronic condition continues, there is usually a decrease or loss of appetite. Decreased activity, weight loss, and/or weakness may occur. Other symptoms of illness will depend on the particular disease process. (For example, with chronic pancreatitis, the pancreas may lose its ability to make insulin; the dog will develop diabetes and all the symptoms associated with that problem.) The most common chronic illnesses in dogs are chronic renal failure (see pages 127-129) and chronic cough (see pages 81-83).

Diagnosis of a chronic illness is usually through an examination, blood testing, and X-rays. Other tests may include ultrasound, endoscopy, and even CT scans and MRI's. Treatment is based on the particular problem; however, there are common guidelines that hold true for all chronic illnesses.

Once a chronic illness is diagnosed, you must communicate effectively with your veterinarian on an ongoing basis. You should report any and all subtle changes in your dog's condition, and let your veterinarian determine which changes are significant. Periodic rechecks are helpful to access any changes. Your veterinarian will prescribe medicines to lessen any complications from the disease. (For example, a potassium deficiency caused by kidney disease is easily treated with a supplement.)

Adjustments in your pet's diet may slow the disease process and lessen the symptoms of the problem. Loss or decrease of appetite is one of the most common side effects of chronic disease. There are some feeding preparation techniques that may benefit your dog. (See pages 167-170.) Food should always be fresh, and any food changes should be introduced gradually to avoid digestive upsets. Dogs with decreased appetites may be encouraged to eat by warming their food to enhance the smell and flavor. Also, the addition of water, bouillon, clam juice or garlic to dry food may make the food more appealing. Additionally, some dogs are more likely to eat better in the presence of other animals due to the threat of competition. Others can benefit from hand feeding or from having the owner stay and talk during feeding time.

Most dogs with medical conditions benefit from being fed several small feedings per day. This helps the digestion of foods, plus it ensures a continual source of energy throughout the day. The smaller meals may also help dogs on diets feel more satisfied.

A veterinarian can also prescribe medicines and certain vitamins to stimulate your dog's appetite. Also, medications and/or vitamins to treat the underlying disease may lead to an increase in appetite by making your dog feel better.

Make sure your dog has plenty of fresh water. To increase your dog's access to water, you may need to place water bowls in different locations so that your dog can obtain water with minimal effort. Fresh water should never be withheld from an older dog, unless it is vomiting or unless you are advised to do so by your veterinarian. Make sure the dog is helped outside to go to the bathroom at least four times per day (or more often if necessary). If your dog suffers from incontinence (inability to control bowel movements or urinations), make sure that the dog is kept clean and dry. If your dog has lost the ability to walk, then the ability to urinate might also be affected. Your veterinarian can teach you how to push gently on the dog's bladder to promote urination.

For any dog with a chronic illness, you should avoid imposing any additional stress. Stress may have adverse effects on your dog's appetite, attitude and overall health. Provide a secure environment by avoiding any major changes in your dog's lifestyle. Stick to a familiar routine. Providing extra attention and affection, including appropriate grooming and/or massage, may make your dog happier.

If the disease process develops to the point where your dog's quality of life has declined substantially, you may consider several options to improve your dog's short-term comfort. In addition to hospitalization, outpatient treatments, and hospice care, the best option for your pet may be discontinuing uncomfortable treatments. Eventually euthanasia may be the most appropriate action.

How to Improve Comfort for a Dog that has a Chronic Illness

A. Report any changes in attitude or health to your veterinarian.

B. Frequent veterinary examinations may be necessary to determine the need to change any treatment to prolong your dog's life and provide comfort.

C. Medications can be used to prevent further deterioration or lessen complications.

D. Fresh water should always be available. Never withhold water from an older dog unless the dog is vomiting or unless you are advised to do so by your veterinarian.

E. Increase access to water by placing several water bowls throughout the house, including where the dog lies.

F. Make sure your dog gets proper nourishment
   1. Nutritional consultation and diet change may be recommended according to your dog's age, weight, medical status, and veterinarian's recommendation.
   2. Make sure your dog's food is fresh.
   3. Feed your dog food that is recommended by your veterinarian. Human food should be used only as a last resort if your dog refuses to eat recommended dog food.
   4. A different diet may increase interest in food, but make sure any dietary changes are made gradually and follow your veterinarian's recommendations.
   5. If your dog is reluctant to eat, try warming the food, or try adding water, bouillon, clam juice, or garlic to enhance the food.
   6. Serving food in the presence of other animals may increase your dog's appetite.
   7. Human companionship through petting and talking may encourage the dog to eat.
   8. Feed your dog several small meals throughout the day.

G. Avoid stressing pets that have cancer or any chronic disease.

H. Help your dog outside to go the bathroom at least four times per day.

I. Keep the dog clean and dry.

COLITIS

Colitis is inflammation of the colon. A dog experiencing colitis may have blood or mucous in its stools. The stools may be soft, dark and/or larger in volume. The dog may strain after or during a bowel movement. If no bowel movement is produced, check under the dog's tail for evidence of soft stool pasted to the hair. The dog may need to go outside often and may express this need in an urgent manner. Colitis has many different causes, including allergic reactions, dietary indiscretions (including nondigestible objects), parasitic infestations and cancers. Aging dogs may be more sensitive to dietary changes that can lead to colitis. Colitis which recurs or is chronic may be a sign that there is a more serious underlying problem. Though not all causes of colitis are serious, the amount of discomfort the dog feels can be great.

The cause of colitis can be determined by a series of tests. A stool specimen should be checked for parasites and clostridia bacteria. Blood tests can be performed to rule out disease processes that could result in colitis. X-rays may be necessary to further examine the bowels. Your veterinarian may perform a colonoscopy, a diagnostic test that uses a flexible fiberoptic scope to look directly at the the inside of the colon. A colonoscopy can also be used to retrieve a biopsy (i.e., a tissue sample for laboratory analysis).

Treatment of colitis should be aimed at treating the underlying cause of the colitis, providing comfort, and preventing recurrences of the condition.

How To Improve Comfort

A. If there is no foreign object protruding from the rectum and there are no signs of illness other than colitis, withhold food for 4 hours. (This time reference is for a normal, otherwise healthy, adult dog. Debilitated older dogs should not be restricted from food for more than a couple of hours.) DO NOT withhold water unless your dog is vomiting. If there are other symptoms of illness, such as vomiting, lack of appetite or listlessness, contact a veterinarian immediately. If your dog has no symptoms of other

77

illness but is not more comfortable within 4 hours, contact a veterinarian.

B. If any foreign object (e.g., grass, string, cloth, etc.) is protruding from the rectum, DO NOT pull on the object; it could lacerate the bowels. Instead, if the object is protruding more than four inches, cut the object with a scissors (to within four inches of the rectum), taking care not to cut the dog. Contact a veterinarian immediately.

C. If there is no vomiting, feed the dog Kaopectate® using an eyedropper or dosage syringe:
    (1) 1 to 2 teaspoons for dogs weighing less than 20 pounds,
    (2) 3 to 4 teaspoons for dogs weighing 20 or more pounds.

D. Repeat Step C every 4 to 6 hours for adult dogs.

E. Add 1-2 teaspoons of bran flakes to your dog's meals to increase the fiber in your pet's diet, or obtain a high-fiber prescription food from your veterinarian.

F. To aid your dog's digestion, feed your dog more frequently but in smaller portions.

G. Many times colitis requires treatment by a veterinarian with antibiotics or anti-inflammatory medications.

CONSTIPATION

Constipation in a dog refers to the inability of the dog to have a bowel movement over a period of a few days. The causes of constipation are numerous. Diet irregularities such as the ingestion of hair, grass, bone, fabric or wood can cause the bowels to become impacted (i.e., blocked). Lack of fiber can be a contributing factor. Certain drugs can slow the bowels or cause hardened stools. Also, any condition that causes your dog pain while pushing to defecate can cause your dog to go too long between bowel movements. (Examples of these conditions include anal sac abscesses, pelvic fractures, back pain, and tumors in the colon.) Enlarged prostate glands or hernias around the rectum may also cause the stool to accumulate, and any illness that causes dehydration may predispose your dog to constipation. Metabolic diseases, such as hypothyroidism, may also have an effect on the bowels. In addition to the fact that spinal cord injuries and degeneration impair the sensations of having bowel movements, these difficulties may make it impossible for your dog to push during a bowel movement.

Regardless of the cause of constipation, many of the symptoms are the same. Straining is usually the hallmark sign. (Note, however, that a dog that strains to have a bowel movement is not necessarily constipated. See Straining on pages 143-145.) If the constipation starts to interfere with the dog's electrolyte balance and causes inflammation inside the colon, other signs of illness may appear, such as vomiting and depression. Often the dog will develop diarrhea while constipated; the diarrhea can pass around the obstruction of the hard stool so the dog can still be constipated even if diarrhea is present. Therefore, it is important not to mistake diarrhea for a successful bowel movement.

Even without any complicating factors, constipation can have serious consequences if not tended to promptly. With constipation, the stool inside becomes harder and drier over time, which makes removal more difficult. The retention of stool can result in lack of appetite, vomiting and dehydration. Prolonged retention of stool can also cause permanent enlargement and nerve damage to the colon.

Any time a bowel movement is not produced within a 48-hour period, consult a veterinarian for help. Usually constipation can be diagnosed with an examination, although determining the cause of the constipation may require testing. A veterinarian can perform blood tests to identify diseases that could cause constipation. In some instances X-rays or a colonoscopy may be necessary to further examine the bowels. (A colonoscopy is a diagnostic test that uses a fiberoptic scope to directly look at the the inside of the colon and retrieve a biopsy.) Once the cause of the constipation has been determined, treatment is directed at curing that problem.

Simple constipation without any complicating factors can be treated most safely by a veterinarian. A series of delicate enemas and sedation may be required to relieve the impaction. Prevention of dehydration is also important to avoid further complications, especially in the aging pet.

There are several precautions that you can take to help prevent problems with constipation. First, make sure that your dog always has an adequate supply of fresh water. Second, consult your veterinarian regarding dietary changes, such as increasing fiber, to help reduce the likelihood of a recurrence of constipation. And third, make sure you walk your dog more often and longer than usual to provide the dog an increased opportunity to have bowel movements.

How to Prevent and/or Relieve Constipation

A. If your dog is uncomfortable or if more than 2 days have passed since your dog's last bowel movement, contact your veterinarian.

B. Ask your veterinarian about an enema for the dog. An enema should be performed by a professional because a dog can be injured easily if it struggles during the process.

C. If your dog has a tendency to become constipated, upon the advice of your veterinarian, practice the following precautions:

    1. Encourage your dog to drink water.

    2. Add 1-2 teaspoons of bran flakes to your dog's meals to increase the fiber in your pet's diet or obtain a high-fiber prescription food from your veterinarian.

    3. To aid your dog's digestion, feed your dog more frequently but in smaller portions.

    4. Add 1/4 teaspoon to 1 teaspoon of metamucil into your dog's food to help soften your dog's stools.

    5. Walk your dog longer and more frequently.

COUGHING

Coughing, a common symptom in aging dogs, is a warning sign of several problems. Coughs can be categorized by their characteristics. A cough may be sporadic or persistent; it may be dry or productive (i.e., bringing up fluid); it may also be acute (i.e., sudden) or chronic (i.e., lasting more than 2 months). By observing the type of cough, you can help your veterinarian with diagnosing the problem and its severity.

Even though older dogs often develop harsh, sudden coughs, these coughs are not normal. The development of a harsh, sudden cough may be caused by infections that lead to tonsillitis, bronchitis, pneumonia, asthma or obstruction of the airways.

With aging dogs, chronic coughs are more common than harsh, sudden coughs. There are four common causes of chronic coughs in dogs: heartworm disease, bronchial disease, tracheal/bronchial collapse, and heart failure. Heartworm disease is a condition whereby worms live in the dog's heart and the blood vessels that enter the lungs. Over time, the condition is usually fatal because the worms cause the heart to fail. The interesting fact about heartworms is that they are transmitted by mosquitoes. A mosquito bites the dog, thereby placing an infective larva in the skin. This larva develops and migrates to the heart over a 2-4 month period. It takes about 2-3 months for the worm to mature and produce its babies (microfilaria) which are released into the blood stream. The babies can then be picked up by mosquitoes and infect other dogs. In the meantime, the adult worms cause severe changes in the heart that can cause secondary problems with the lungs, liver, and kidneys. Heartworm disease in dogs is preventable. A once-a-month preventive medicine is available for dogs, or there is a six-month injectable that can be used instead. This preventive medicine can be obtained from your veterinarian. If a dog is unfortunate enough to contract the disease, it is treatable through a series of injections and oral medicines. Every dog that lives in a heartworm region should be given a blood test once per year to check for the disease, regardless of whether the dog has been taking heartworm preventive medicine all year. The test is necessary because the medicine is not always 100% effective.

Chronic bronchial disease is a problem that affects older dogs, usually those over the age of eight. Smaller breeds, especially

81

poodles, Shetland sheepdogs, Pomeranians, Pekingese, Chihuahuas and Yorkshire terriers, more frequently contract the disease. Chronic bronchitis is a disease of the bronchioles (i.e., the small airways of the lungs). The airways may be irritated from a number of causes, such as infection, allergies and/or parasites. Diagnosis is generally made through physical examination, chest X-rays and blood tests. Additional testing, such as a tracheal wash or bronchoscopy, may be required to determine the specific cause. Treatment is based on curing the problem plus lessening the discomfort caused by the cough.

Tracheal (wind pipe) and bronchiolar collapse occur in middle-aged to older dogs. Smaller breeds, such as Chihuahuas, toy poodles, Pomeranians, Shih Tzus, Lhasa apsos, and Yorkshire terriers, are affected most often. The condition develops when the rings of the trachea lose their rigidity and become flaccid. This is further complicated if there is increased pressure applied to the chest from lifting the dog, or increased pressure from internal fat or heart enlargement applying pressure to the bronchioles. Dogs with collapsing tracheas may have a dry, honking cough that gets progressively worse. The cough may start gradually, perhaps appearing only when the dog gets excited, but eventually the cough becomes more prevalent and occurs even when the dog is resting. The cough is the dog's way of popping open the airway that has collapsed. Diagnosis is usually through examinations and X-rays. Treatment must be directed toward the underlying cause (e.g., obesity, heart difficulties, etc.) and may include decreasing weight in obese dogs, treating any heart condition, and/or prescribing bronchodilators and cough suppressants.

Chronic cough is a typical early sign of heart disease. The cough may originate because an enlarged heart is exerting pressure on the windpipe making it difficult to breathe, or the cough may result from fluid collecting in the lungs (because of an inefficient heart and changes in blood pressure). Because a cough may be the first warning sign of a heart problem, do not ignore it. Early treatment for a heart condition may greatly improve your dog's chances of a good outcome.

Less common, but increasing in prevalence as a dog ages, is a cough caused by the aspiration of food into the airway passages. As a dog becomes older, the nerves and muscles of the throat and esophagus may degenerate making swallowing and the passage of food more difficult. Sometimes this food enters the airways causing irritation and pneumonia.

Cough is often a warning sign of a more serious problem. If your dog develops a cough, make sure the pet gets immediate veterinary attention to ascertain the exact nature of the difficulty and to treat it appropriately.

How to Improve Comfort

A. Avoid all stress. The least amount of stress may precipitate a crisis if your dog cannot breathe properly.
B. Plan the handling and activities of your dog to minimize excitement. Never hold your dog tightly.
C. If the dog appears to be in a crisis, keep your dog in an upright position (i.e., belly down). Never lay your dog on its back or side because those positions make breathing more difficult by putting extra pressure on the chest.
D. If the cough persists, see a veterinarian as soon as possible. Note whether the cough is dry or productive so that your veterinarian can better advise you regarding additional treatment.
E. If the cause of the cough is unknown, offer the pet 1/4 cup of prepared chicken bouillon to soothe the throat while waiting to get help from your veterinarian.

CUSHING'S DISEASE

Cushing's disease (hyperadrenocorticism) is a condition in which a dog produces too much cortisol. Cortisol is a hormone that is produced in the dog's adrenal gland. Overproduction of cortisol can occur when either the pituitary gland or adrenal glands malfunction. In some cases, these malfunctions are caused by benign or malignant tumors on these glands. While cortisol is essential for the dog, too much will cause substantial health problems. Early symptoms of Cushing's disease include increased thirst, frequent urination, panting, hair loss, skin infections, hardened areas on the skin, overall thinning of the skin, enlarged abdomen, black heads, increased appetite, increased weight gain, and sometimes heart conditions. Although dogs that are middle-aged or older are more susceptible to Cushing's disease, the condition can occur in dogs as young as three years old. Breeds that are at higher risk include silky terriers, bull terriers, Boston terriers, Yorkshire terriers, dachshunds, and all types of poodles.

Diagnosis of Cushing's disease is made by a combination of physical findings, urine tests, blood tests, and ultrasound. The information gathered by these tests helps determine whether the excess cortisol is being produced by a problem in the pituitary gland versus the adrenal gland. Your veterinarian will need to find the origin of the Cushing's disease in order to provide proper treatment. The following five tests are commonly used in the diagnosis process:

Urine Cortisol to Creatinine Ratio Test – This test detects the amount of cortisol appearing in the urine. This test is the screening test for Cushing's disease (i.e., it is the test to determine whether your dog has the disease). If this test is negative, then your dog does not have Cushing's disease, and no further Cushing's disease tests are necessary. If the test is positive (i.e., if the test indicates a high amount of cortisol in the urine) your dog may have Cushing's disease, and additional testing (described below) is required to determine whether the disease does in fact exist and, if so, to determine the cause of the disease.

ACTH Stimulation Test – This test requires sampling the blood both before and after administration of a drug which tests the body's ability to produce cortisol. The time interval between the first and

84

second blood samples should be one to two hours. This test is used to make the diagnosis of Cushing's disease and to monitor the dog's therapy during treatment. No one test is 100% determinative of the presence of Cushing's disease; therefore, the next test is often used in combination with the ACTH stimulation test.

Low Dose Dexamethasone Suppression Test – This test requires the sampling of blood before, and then two times after, the administration of a low dose of dexamethasone. It takes approximately eight hours to perform from start to finish. Like the ACTH stimulation test, this test is also used to diagnose Cushing's disease. Because no one test is 100% determinative of the presence of Cushing's disease, this test is often used in combination with the ACTH stimulation test.

High Dose Dexamethasone Suppression Test – If the above-described tests indicate the presence of Cushing's disease, then the high dose dexamethasone suppression test is used to indicate whether the cause of the Cushing's disease is malfunction of the pituitary gland versus the adrenal gland. Proper identification of the cause of the Cushing's disease is necessary to determine appropriate treatment options for your pet. One blood test is collected before a high dose of dexamethasone is given, and two more blood samples are collected at later times. This test takes approximately eight hours to perform from start to finish.

Abdominal Ultrasound – While the high dose dexamethasone suppression test is highly effective as a diagnostic tool, the abdominal ultrasound is generally recommended as an additional test of adrenal gland health. This test evaluates the size and shape of the adrenal glands and may indicate the presence of a tumor affecting the glands.

Treatment for Cushing's disease involves decreasing the amount of excess cortisol the dog is manufacturing. If the dog has a tumor on one or both adrenal glands, surgery may be curative. If the dog has overproduction of cortisol from pituitary malfunction, medication can be given to control the disease. If the excess cortisol is the result of adrenal gland dysfunction, medication may be used to selectively destroy portions of the adrenal gland. (Note: overdose from these medications may be life-threatening. Your dog should be observed closely for overdose signs, including loss of appetite, weakness, vomiting, diarrhea and/or collapse. Contact your veterinarian immediately if you suspect you dog is experiencing an overdose.)

The prognosis for a dog with Cushing's disease depends upon the cause, the dog's age, and the dog's overall health. Some dogs may have a shortened life expectancy. Dogs that have Cushing's disease and are not treated may develop life-threatening complications. Regardless of your dog's prognosis, there are ways that you can make your dog more comfortable and help prevent complications. Refer to the outline below.

How to Improve Comfort

A.   Report any unusual signs to your veterinarian. Early signs include increased thirst, urinating in the house, hair loss, enlarged abdomen and increased appetite.

B.   Use all medications as prescribed by the veterinarian.

C.   When administering medications, do not deviate from the dosage or the time interval specified on the label.

D.   When your dog is on medications, report any side effects (e.g., loss of appetite, lethargy, weakness, vomiting and/or diarrhea) to your veterinarian immediately. Some dogs may have severe reactions that can be life threatening, and these dogs may need additional medications to counter these problems.

E.   Follow-up care is mandatory for successful treatment.

F.   If the signs of Cushing's disease return while your dog is on medication, inform your veterinarian of these changes.

G.   Ensure that your dog has easy access to food and water. If your dog has limited mobility, place food and water in more than one location.

H.   If your dog has limited mobility, do not wait for the pet to ask to go outside. Make sure you take your dog outside regularly to prevent broken house habits.

I.   Never punish your dog for broken house habits. Punishment for broken house habits that are medically related can lead to anxiety and additional problems.

DENTAL DISEASE

Dental-related difficulties are a major cause of health problems and discomfort in older dogs. Most dental problems can be avoided by providing your dog with regular veterinary dental care. Dental disease can cause pain and infection and can make your dog seriously ill. Even though dogs feel pain, they may not exhibit it by their actions. Infection that starts as dental disease can spread into the bloodstream where it can cause a variety of problems, including damage to the heart, liver and kidneys and ultimately death.

The most common dental disorder in aging dogs is periodontal disease. Periodontal disease refers to problems occurring in the tissues surrounding the teeth, such as the gums (gingiva), other connective tissues, and bone. It may occur in four stages of varying degrees of severity. At stage one there is redness around the tooth at the gum line accompanied by a small amount of plaque (a film of bacteria, food, saliva, and debris) on the tooth. At stage two the gums become more inflamed and begin to swell. There is an increased build-up of plaque and calculus (a hard, mineralization of plaque). The third stage involves the pocketing of the gum around the tooth plus more build-up of plaque and calculus. In the final fourth stage the disease is advanced, and there is severe inflammation accompanied by receding gums and deeper pocket formation. The pockets fill with pus, and the bone surrounding the teeth deteriorates. Even in mild cases, the presence of infection in the mouth poses great risk to the dog.

Another common and serious dental disorder is called an abscess. Abscesses of the tooth root occur more commonly in older dogs. An abscess is caused when infection develops around the tooth, sometimes from a crack in the tooth. The signs of an abscess include one or more of the following; swelling below the eyes, pawing at the mouth, difficulty chewing, avoiding hard dog food, teeth chattering and/or drooling. Treatment usually involves a root canal or extraction of the tooth in combination with antibiotic therapy.

An aging dog is susceptible to a variety of dental and mouth problems, including oral tumors, polyps (epulides), and overgrowth of gums. A dog's mouth should be closely examined for any changes, not just those on the teeth. As part of your dog's routine physical examination, your veterinarian should check the back of your dog's throat, as well as under the tongue. The most common malignancies in a dog's mouth are malignant melanoma and squamous cell carcinomas. Report any changes such as bad breath, lumps, loose teeth, face deformities, drooling and/or difficulty chewing, immediately to your veterinarian.

Worn teeth are a common occurrence in aging dogs, especially among those that are frequent chewers. A worn tooth that loses the enamel over a period of time will have a protective layer of dentin (a substance harder than bone) covering the pulp (nerves and blood supply) of the tooth. This protective layer of dentin will help prevent the tooth from becoming diseased. Worn teeth usually pose no discomfort or health risk when the changes have occurred slowly. Your doctor will be able to assess whether your dog's worn teeth are a problem.

In order to prevent, diagnose and treat dental problems, your veterinarian may recommend regular dental cleanings based on your dog's needs. Many conditions are difficult to see in the dog's mouth while the pet is awake and many dental conditions cannot be discovered without the use of oral X-rays. Cleaning a dog's teeth (a dental prophy) is performed under anesthesia. Precautions are taken to make sure that the dog's risk is minimized. (See pages 208-210.) Routine dental procedures take a minimum of forty five minutes to perform. Often there are new findings of dental problems uncovered during a routine cleaning that require immediate attention and additional time. One example would be treating deep pockets between the tooth and gum (periodontal disease). By performing root planing or curettage to remove plaque from the roots so the tissues can heal, or applying a special long-acting antibiotic deep into the tissues, many diseased teeth can be saved.

There are 10 steps to the dental cleaning and examination:
1. Preliminary exam of oral cavity, including tonsils, hard and soft palate, and under tongue.
2. Application of antiseptic in mouth.
3. Removal of plaque and calculus above the gum line.
4. Removal of plaque and calculus below the gum line.
5. Application of disclosing solution to check for hidden plaque.
6. Thorough exam and charting of dental problems.
7. Oral X-rays (radiographs) of teeth and jaw.
8. Teeth polishing.
9. Fluoride treatment.
10. Thorough rinsing and application of antiseptic gel.

Between veterinary visits, you should watch for a number of warning signs, including gum redness, bleeding gums, bad breath, drooling, painful chewing, plaque build up, sneezing, lumps, facial deformities, and excess nasal discharge. Report any of these signs to your dog's veterinarian.

Home dental care may help decrease the risk of your dog developing serious dental problems and may decrease the need for expensive and painful dental procedures. Because each dog is an individual, and some are more willing to have their mouth worked on than others, a home dental program must be tailored for your specific dog. The following guidelines should provide a foundation to help design a program that is right for your pet.

First, you must consider your dog's general temperament and attitude. While some dogs will allow their owner to handle them in any way ranging from cleaning their ears to performing toenail trims, other dogs will not even tolerate having their hair brushed. The latter type of dog might not allow you to perform any type of home dental care. If there is any concern that your dog may bite, do not attempt dental care at home.

An older dog that has never had its mouth manipulated can be trained like a puppy. Start by rubbing your dog's face, working your way toward the mouth. You should praise your dog for holding still while you are doing this. Repeat this procedure several times a day until your pet is used to it and does not pull away. Next, while rubbing your dog's mouth, focus on touching and gently lifting the lips. Praise your dog for holding still, and repeat this technique several times a day. Once your dog is used to this, show your dog the toothbrush or applicator for applying the dental care product, and rub it on the outside of your dog's mouth. Repeat this until your dog is comfortable with the object being in the general area of its mouth. The next step involves lifting the lips and touching the toothbrush or applicator to the teeth and gums. As before, repeat this until your dog is comfortable with it. When your dog readily accepts these procedures, a small portion of hygiene paste, solution or gel may be used. Increase the portion of paste, solution, or gel once your dog is comfortable with the original volume. Depending on the dog, each of these steps may take several minutes or several days to perfect. Remember to reward your dog with a treat after each success. For the greatest effectiveness, home dental hygiene should be practiced every day.

There are many dental products available on the market for dogs. Besides a variety of pastes, sprays or solutions and gels, there are enzyme-coated rawhide chews and dental-exercise toys. The pastes, sprays, solutions and gels are meant to be applied to the teeth by using a pet or child's toothbrush, finger toothbrush, gauze sponge, or cotton applicator. The pastes are probably the most palatable for your dog. Pastes come in a variety of flavors, including malt and poultry flavors. Never use human pastes because they foam too much for dogs and can cause problems if swallowed.

Dental care at home should be performed daily. When you are brushing your dog's teeth, make sure you brush all of the teeth. When brushing or wiping solutions on the teeth, brush or wipe away from the gum line. Also, the insides of the teeth should ideally be cleaned, but many dogs will not tolerate it, and you may risk being bitten. Luckily, the insides of the teeth are usually less affected by plaque than the outer surfaces. Because of the risk of being bitten, before deciding to clean the inner surfaces of your dog's teeth, consult with your veterinarian.

If brushing your dog's teeth is not a viable option for your dog or for you, then you should consider either a special dental rawhide chew with enzymes, a dental-care toy, and/or a hygiene solution mixed into the pet's drinking water. The rawhide chews with enzymes allow your dog to do the work; when the dog chews, the dog's mouth is exposed to the enzymes which break down plaque. With a dental-care toy, you will achieve similar results. The dental-care toys may be filled with dog toothpaste, and when the dog chews, the paste is released onto the dog's teeth. Your veterinarian can help you make the decision about which home dental-hygiene method is best for your dog.

Report any changes in your dog's mouth to your veterinarian. In particular, report any reddened or bleeding gums, calculus buildup on the teeth, any pus, sore gums, bad breath, lump or bump in the mouth, and any loose teeth. If the gums bleed after brushing, consult your veterinarian before continuing with home dental care.

How to Promote Proper Dental Care

A. Have your dog's teeth checked at least twice each year by a veterinarian.

B. Between veterinary visits, report any gum redness, bleeding gums, bad breath, drooling, painful chewing, plaque build up, sneezing, lumps, facial deformities, and excess nasal discharge to your veterinarian.

C. Perform dental hygiene at home on a daily basis.

    1. Choose a paste, solution or spray, or gel recommended by your veterinarian for dental hygiene.

    2. Choose a child's tooth brush, pet tooth brush, finger toothbrush, gauze sponge, or cotton tipped applicator.

    3. Gradually accustom your dog to having its mouth handled gradually; then slowly introduce the mechanical devices to your dog. Once your dog is used to those, apply small quantities of the paste, solution, or gel to the teeth.

    4. If your dog will not tolerate having its mouth handled, choose enzyme-covered rawhide chews, a dental exerciser toy, and/or a hygiene solution mixed into the pet's drinking water.

    5. Use products daily.

    6. If the gums bleed after home dental care, consult your veterinarian before continuing.

D. Follow your veterinarian's advice for scheduling dental visits.

DIABETES

Diabetes in dogs usually occurs between the age of seven to nine, but it can be seen earlier. Female dogs are more prone to the disease, as are some breeds. Cairn terriers, miniature pinschers, toy poodles, dachshunds, miniature schnauzers, and beagles are at higher risk. Dogs that are obese and/or have been afflicted with pancreatitis may also be more prone to developing the disease.

Diabetes is a disease in which the body (specifically the pancreas) does not produce enough insulin (the substance that processes sugar in the bloodstream). Diabetes is a disease that makes the body unable to use the sugar in the blood for energy, thereby causing the blood sugar level to be abnormally high. In a dog suffering from diabetes, the sugar in the blood is so high that some of it ends up being processed into the urine. When the body cannot use its usual energy source (sugar), the body starts to use other sources of energy, such as fat and protein from muscle. This breakdown and utilization of fat may have serious consequences because insulin is also necessary for its proper metabolism. The improper metabolism of fat causes waste products that can make the dog extremely sick; this condition is called ketosis.

The first symptoms of diabetes usually include increased urination and thirst. Depression, confusion, cataracts, vomiting, diarrhea, weight loss, and sometimes weight gain are other symptoms that can occur. Diagnosis of diabetes is accomplished through urine and blood tests.

While there is no cure for diabetes, there is a treatment that reduces the detrimental effects. Insulin injections take some of the sugar from the blood and make it available for the dog's body to use for energy so that the dog's system is not trying to process fat and proteins for energy. By making sugar available for energy, via the use of insulin, and lowering the level of sugar in the blood, the signs of diabetes typically lessen. To ensure that your dog receives the proper dosage of insulin, your pet will need to spend time in the hospital while treatment of insulin is initiated. Your pet will be monitored for reaction to the dose and will be monitored for side effects and, if necessary, treated for diabetes complications.

Even though learning to treat diabetes is easy with practice, it may be stressful at the beginning. Follow your veterinarian's instructions closely, and ask questions about anything you might not understand.

Giving your dog injections is easy to learn. Practice by injecting water into an orange. The sensation of sticking an orange is similar to sticking a dog, in terms of surface resistance to the needle. When you do give your dog an injection, make sure that there are no bubbles in the insulin syringe. Have your veterinarian demonstrate the technique for removing bubbles. Give the injections under the loose skin between the shoulder blades. Reward your dog with praise or a treat before and after the injection. If you have tried to administer an injection but you are not sure whether the insulin actually went into the dog (as opposed to onto its hair), DO NOT repeat the injection. Overdose can be fatal. Always store insulin in the refrigerator.

Your dog's progress will be monitored via a glucose curve, a diagnostic aid that consists of a series of blood tests taken over a relatively short period of time (one day or less). In addition, your veterinarian may run a test to monitor your dog's fructosamine level. These tests will help your veterinarian determine the need for insulin dosage adjustment.

In addition to insulin injections, controlling weight, maintaining proper diet and exercising are important parts of diabetes treatment. Overweight pets typically do not respond to insulin as well as more fit pets. Therefore, if your dog is overweight and has diabetes, you should discuss a weight-loss plan with your veterinarian. Also note that underweight dogs should be brought up to optimal weight to help in regulating their sugar. Regardless of whether your dog needs to lose weight or gain weight, the type of diet that is best tolerated by diabetic dogs is a diet balanced in carbohydrates and high in fiber. Increased fiber makes digestion occur more evenly, making regulation easier. Semi-moist foods should be avoided because they tend to be high in simple sugars and cause great swings in sugar levels after eating. Canned or dry foods are preferred. Ask your veterinarian which particular food may be best for your dog.

Dogs receiving a once-a-day injection of insulin should be fed three times daily. One meal should be given at the time of the injection, another 6-8 hours after the injection, and a third meal about 6-8 hours later. If twice-a-day insulin is given, the dog should be fed four times per day: a meal at each insulin injection and a meal six hours after each injection. If your dog does not eat after its injection, watch for low blood sugar side effects, such as weakness, disorientation, seizures, or coma. If you notice any of these side effects, contact your veterinarian immediately.

In addition to proper, regulated feedings, there are other steps that can be taken to promote the benefits of insulin treatments. Keeping your dog's exercise level relatively constant will help decrease fluctuations in insulin requirements. Keeping your dog healthy with proper medical care and periodic physical examinations will help your pet to cope with the effects of diabetes. Also note that spayed or neutered dogs have less difficulty with hormones affecting the insulin treatment.

One of the most serious complications that can result from treating diabetics can occur when the sugar in the blood falls too low after administering insulin. Some of the signs of low blood sugar include weakness, disorientation, seizure, or coma. If you observe any of these symptoms in a diabetic dog and the dog is conscious, feed the dog one teaspoon of corn syrup. If corn syrup is not available, then substitute with honey or maple syrup. DO NOT feed the dog any chocolate because chocolate is toxic to dogs. If the dog is in a coma, rub the corn syrup on the dog's gums. Contact a veterinarian immediately.

It is important to consult your doctor with any questions or concerns you may have about the treatment of diabetes.

Diagnosing and Treating Diabetes

A. If your dog is consuming an increased amount of water or if the dog is urinating large quantities, have the dog checked for diabetes.

B. If your dog is diagnosed with diabetes, control the dog's weight, monitor the dog's diet and exercise the dog regularly as recommended by a veterinarian.

C. Never feed a diabetic dog semi-moist feeds. Instead, feed your pet canned or dry foods balanced in carbohydrates and high in fiber. Ask your veterinarian.

D. Consult with your veterinarian regarding the benefits of having the dog spayed or neutered.

E. If any unusual signs develop or if the symptoms of diabetes return after treatment begins, call your veterinarian.

F. If weakness, disorientation, seizures, or coma occur after insulin is given, administer 1 teaspoon of corn syrup (or honey or maple syrup) orally. If your dog is unconscious, rub the syrup on its gums. Contact a veterinarian immediately.

DIARRHEA OR SOFT STOOLS

It is not normal for a dog to have soft stools or diarrhea. Pets can have diarrhea without showing other signs of illness, yet the situation can be serious. If diarrhea persists without treatment, your dog could suffer complications, including malnutrition from improper absorption of nutrients, dehydration, and anemia from slow loss of small quantities of blood from bowel irritation.

There are many causes of diarrhea in a dog. Diarrhea or soft stools may be caused by dietary indiscretions, infections, inflammation, obstructions, parasites or exposure to toxins. Older dogs are at higher risk of many additional causes of diarrhea, such as intolerance to certain drugs, digestive ulceration, diabetes, kidney disease, liver disease, electrolyte imbalances, cancers, constipation, pancreatitis, and other metabolic problems.

If your dog has soft stools, there are some observations you should make to help your veterinarian obtain a proper diagnosis of the origin of the problem. First, note the consistency of the stools (i.e., soft versus watery). Next, note whether there is any blood or mucous in the stool. Is the stool tarry (i.e., darkened by the presence of blood)? Finally, note whether your dog is passing a large quantity or a relatively small quantity of fecal matter.

In addition to the observations that you make, your veterinarian will want a stool sample for examination under a microscope and for other tests. The examination of the stool under the microscope will enable the veterinarian to identify whether there are any parasites that might be the cause of the problem. In addition, your veterinarian may perform other stool tests and blood tests to rule out disease processes that could result in diarrhea. Depending upon the situation, other tests may be advisable. For example, X-rays may be necessary to further examine the bowels. If there is reason to suspect underlying disease processes, such as cancer or inflammatory bowel disease, your veterinarian may recommend a colonoscopy or endoscopy, a diagnostic test that uses a flexible fiberoptic scope to directly look at the inside of the bowels and retrieve a biopsy (i.e., a tissue sample to be analyzed by a lab).

Treatment for diarrhea must be aimed at treating the cause of the diarrhea, providing comfort and preventing recurrence of the condition.

Diagnosis and Treatment of Diarrhea

A. Note the frequency and substance of the diarrhea.

B. Your veterinarian may request a stool sample for examination under the microscope (to check for intestinal parasites) and to run other tests.

C. Proper diagnosis and medication from your veterinarian can prevent serious side effects from the diarrhea.

D. If there is no foreign object protruding from the rectum and there are no signs of illness other than diarrhea, withhold food for 4 hours. (This time recommendation is for a normal, otherwise healthy, adult dog. Debilitated older dogs should not be restricted from food for more than a couple of hours.) DO NOT withhold water unless your dog is vomiting. If there are other symptoms of illness, such as vomiting, lack of appetite or listlessness, contact a veterinarian immediately. If your dog has no symptoms of other illness but is not more comfortable within 4 hours, contact a veterinarian. Many times diarrhea requires treatment with antibiotics or anti-inflammatory drugs.

E. If any foreign object (e.g., grass, string, cloth, etc.) is protruding from the rectum, do not pull on the object; it could lacerate the bowels. Instead, if the object is protruding more than four inches, cut the object with a scissors (to within four inches of the rectum) taking care not to cut the dog. Contact a veterinarian immediately.

F. If there is no vomiting, feed the dog Kaopectate® using an eyedropper or dosage syringe:
   (1) 1 to 2 teaspoons for dogs weighing less than 20 pounds,
   (2) 3 to 4 teaspoons for dogs weighing 20 or more pounds.

G. Repeat Step F every 4 to 6 hours for an adult dog until symptoms disappear. But if symptoms have not disappeared within 4 hours, consult your veterinarian.

H. Add 1-2 teaspoons of bran flakes to your dog's meals to increase the fiber in your pet's regular diet.

I.   To aid your dog's digestion, feed your dog more frequently but in smaller portions.

J.   When you do resume feeding your dog, the best home remedy for diarrhea is to prepare a 50/50 mixture of boiled hamburger (drain off the water and fat) and plain cooked rice. Appropriate feedings are as follows:
(1) 1/4 cup of the mixture 4 times per day for small dogs,
(2) 1/2 cup of the mixture 4 times per day for medium dogs,
(3) 3/4 cup of the mixture 4 times per day for large dogs.
Your veterinarian may wish to adjust the servings or may recommend a prescription diet instead.

K.   If symptoms persist for more than 4 hours, or if they worsen or return, contact your veterinarian immediately.

L.   If your dog has other signs along with the diarrhea (e.g., vomiting, loss of coordination, fatigue, etc.) contact a veterinarian.

M.   Because some infections can be transmitted to people, wash your hands after handling your dog or cleaning up accidents.

DIFFICULTY GETTING UP

Aging dogs may be slow at getting up and moving around. There are several common causes of this problem, including osteoarthritis, neck and back pain, nerve degeneration, and weakness from other diseases.

Osteoarthritis or degenerative joint disease is common in the aging dog. Osteoarthritis occurs when the cartilage lining the joint surface breaks down and bone is deposited in the joint. As a joint ages, the cartilage lining the joint changes in its chemical makeup and becomes more easily damaged. The degenerative joint disease in dogs usually occurs from three sources: (1) normal aging changes of the joint surfaces, (2) damage to the joint from a previous injury, and/or (3) developmental problems such as hip dysplasia (poorly developed hip joint) or patellar luxations (slipping of the knee cap).

The signs of osteoarthritis include stiffness (especially after resting for long periods or after extended exercise), reluctance to rise, hesitation in climbing or jumping, and crying when moving. Physical changes include loss of muscle tone, loss of muscle mass of affected area, swelling over the affected joint and/or pain over the affected joint. Diagnosis is usually through a thorough physical examination and X-rays.

The area of the dog's body most commonly affected by degenerative joint disease is the hind end. When the hind end is affected, the dog experiences difficulty rising from a sitting or lying position.

Degenerative joint disease along the spine is referred to as spondylosis. Spondylosis is common in older dogs, especially older large breeds, and is particularly common in boxers, Labradors and German shepherds. With spondylosis, bone spurs develop on the vertebrae, sometimes fusing the spine together. The bony growth may compress nerves, making it hard for the dog to get up. Some dogs will walk with an exaggerated arched or straight back.

Back and neck pain may also be the result of a muscle strain, trauma or a variety of other difficulties, including arthritis or even a tumor near the spine. In some instances the injury may be a herniated (i.e., slipped) disc.

Disc disease in dogs causes a variety of symptoms depending upon the location and severity of the condition. When a disc "slips" out of place or herniates, it applies pressure to the spinal cord or nerves leading from the cord, creating the pain or paralysis. Symptoms may range from mild neck or back pain to extreme pain or paralysis. Sometimes the pain may radiate down the legs mimicking a lameness. There may be a reluctance to move or participate in routine activities, including hesitation to jump or climb. The dog may cry when petted or lifted. A dog with a herniated disc may also have difficulty lifting its head, making eating difficult. The afflicted dog may hunch its back while walking, fold its toes under, or drag its legs. The dog's bowel movements and urinations may be painful. Because mild cases can quickly worsen into paralysis, prompt veterinary care is essential.

Nerve injury, or more commonly nerve degeneration, can also be a cause of difficulty getting up. Degenerative myelopathy is a nerve disorder that affects large breed dogs, most commonly German shepherds. The symptoms include weakness and loss of coordination in the rear legs. Often the toes of the hind legs will knuckle under and scrape on the ground. Loss of control of the dog's bowels and urinations also can be present. Unfortunately, there is no treatment for this disorder; it usually gets progressively worse with time.

Weakness from disease processes can make it difficult for your dog to get around. Watch for sudden difficulty getting up, loss of appetite, vomiting, diarrhea, weight loss, weight gain, confusion, staggering, and/or coughing. If any signs of illness are associated with difficulty getting up, notify your veterinarian.

There are many ways to help keep your dog comfortable when it has difficulty getting up. First, make sure you keep your dog clean. Good hygiene is one of the most important ways to help care for your dog. Urine can cause urine scald, a severe inflammation of the skin. This painful condition can result in infection. It hastens the development of skin ulcers on dogs that have difficulty getting up.

Providing appropriate bedding for dogs as they age is extremely important. When a dog has difficulty getting up, it is often forced to lie on whatever surface is available, regardless of whether it is comfortable. An uncomfortable surface can exacerbate the problem by making the dog even more stiff. Therefore, provide a padded, insulated surface in a location convenient for your dog. Soft padding is important to prevent bed sores from developing, and insulation is important because cold floors promote stiffness.

The most important feature of a good bed is cleanliness, and any bedding material that you select should therefore be easy to wash. Examples of good bedding include folded comforters, commercial stuffed beds with removable, waterproof covers, or rubber mats covered with a blanket or towels. Foam and similar absorbent materials should be avoided unless a waterproof covering is available. Waterbeds, though easy to clean, need to be large enough for comfort and carefully monitored for proper temperature. The dog's bed should be big enough to allow the dog to stretch out and lie flat. The proper thickness of a bed depends upon the type of material used, but it should be thick enough to provide adequate padding and insulation from the floor. However, the bed should not be too thick nor too high because you want to make sure the dog does not have difficulty getting onto or off of the bedding.

Note that a dog's bed should be situated in a draft free, dry, well-ventilated area. This area should be in a well-supervised part of the house so that you can interact with and observe your dog. Try to avoid dark, damp basements. Place your dog's food and water near the bedding so that there is easy access.

Some owners prefer that their dog sleep in bed with them, but sometimes a dog loses the ability to get into bed because of decreased ability to jump. One solution is to build a ramp out of plywood. The ramp should be at a low angle (e.g., three or four times longer than it is high), and the ramp should have rails on both sides that the dog can balance against, if necessary. Smaller dogs may be lifted into or out of bed. Some dogs may benefit from having a stepping stool near the bed.

Proper footing is an important concept for dogs which have difficulty getting up and down. Slippery floors are hazardous for older dogs who cannot get the necessary traction. Provide the dog with a good surface by using non-skid throw rugs, bath mats or industrial rubber mats. Towels and blankets are soft but too slippery to be of aid.

The most common area of lameness for an older dog is in its hind end. This problem may occur because of arthritis pain or from weakness due to illness or nerve degeneration. While smaller dogs may be lifted and carried where they need to go, medium and large size breeds pose more of a challenge. To help a dog rise that has some strength left in the rear quarters and good front end strength, place a towel under the dog's abdomen. Once the towel is in place, use it as a sling and lift holding both ends with equal pressure. See page 161. To help a dog up that has weak front end and back end strength, place one towel between the front legs and another under the dog's abdomen. Lift the front towel first using equal pressure on both ends of the towel. Once the front end is almost up, start to lift

101

the back towel. A cloth log carrier may be substituted for the towels. When using either towel method, the dog is depending on you for its balance; be careful the dog does not stumble and hit its nose on the ground.

Dogs with front end difficulties can be helped up by running a towel between the front legs then lifting with equal pressure. This method may be facilitated by grasping and gently pulling up on the collar at the same time. See page 163. By helping your dog as it tries to get up and walk, you can help preserve the dog's muscle strength, improve its circulation, and provide ample opportunity for the dog to go outside to go to the bathroom.

To lift and move a medium sized to large dog that does not have the strength to help, put one arm under the dog's stomach (below the ribs) and the other hand under the dog's neck (with the dog's neck in the corner of your elbow). When lifting the dog, bend your knees and lift with equal pressure on both arms. If your strength does not permit you to lift the dog, tuck a blanket under the dog or roll the dog onto a blanket and pull the dog on the blanket or have someone lift opposite corners.

Even though most joint problems are characterized by difficulty getting up, some dogs have difficulty lying down. When this occurs, it is usually because there is an arthritic condition that causes pain. These dogs benefit from you helping them tuck their back legs underneath them. They may also benefit from having something to brace against when trying to lie down, such as the support of your legs. Placing large soft pillows around the dog may allow for a graduated transition from the up to the down position.

The most important factor in keeping an arthritic dog comfortable is proper exercise and weight control. This also applies to dogs with most other joint problems. Compared to a fit dog, an overweight dog will have more difficulty supporting its weight on sore joints. The only time a dog with arthritis should require strict rest is when there is a suddenly painful spell. Most commonly, pain control is managed with anti-inflammatory drugs. Newer anti-inflammatory drugs are more effective with fewer side effects than the older preparations. However, drug therapy is secondary to weight control and exercise. Nutritional supplements, such as glucosamine and chondroitin sulfate, might also be of benefit. Ask your veterinarian.

NOTE: No medications should be given to a dog without consulting your veterinarian. Unprescribed medicines may mask the discomfort that may help the veterinarian make a diagnosis, and many common people medications are harmful to a dog's health.

WARNING: Tylenol® (acetaminophen), Advil® (ibuprofen) and Motrin® (ibuprofen) are toxic to dogs. Tylenol® cannot be metabolized by the liver and may result in liver failure. Liver failure may be preceded by weakness, blue gums, difficulty breathing, vomiting, diarrhea, and/or the presence of dark urine. Ibuprofen causes severe stomach ulcers and sometimes liver and kidney disease; symptoms include vomiting, diarrhea, listlessness, increased thirst, and/or increased urinations.

Contact your veterinarian if there is any change in your dog's ability to get up and down or if you need advise on the best ways to provide for your dog's mobility, care and comfort.

How to Treat and Transport

A. When symptoms appear (i.e., when you notice your dog is having difficulty getting up or otherwise appears to be suffering from neck or back pain):

1. Contact your veterinarian.
2. Keep the dog quiet and restrict all activity.

B. Comfort and treatment:

1. If the dog has not sustained an injury but rather has a chronic condition, such as arthritis, gentle massage along the dog's neck and back may help relax muscles, if the dog will allow it.
2. If the dog is having difficulty getting up because of arthritis, a special exercise plan will help keep your dog's muscles toned. See pages 45-48.
3. Restrict activity only if a sudden painful event occurs.
4. If your dog suffers from arthritis, ask your veterinarian about certain supplements that may help decrease damage to cartilage.
5. Depending upon your dog's condition, your veterinarian may recommend certain medicines to help control pain.
6. If your dog has difficulty going up and down steps, build a ramp. Make sure the slope is gentle (i.e., 4 feet of length for every 1 foot of height).
7. A towel or cloth log placed under your dog's abdomen can

be used to help lift your dog when the pet is having trouble raising its hind quarters. See page 161.

C. Bedding and food:
   1. Keep all bedding clean.
   2. Provide a soft bed large enough for the dog to lie flat.
   3. Locate the bed in a draft-free, dry, well-ventilated environment.
   4. Locate the dog's bed where the dog can be closely monitored.
   5. Keep food and water in close proximity.
   6. If your dog has difficulty getting up and is overweight, start a weight reduction plan under the guidance of a veterinarian. Your veterinarian may recommend foods that are high in fiber and relatively low in calories.
   7. If your dog is having difficulty bending down to reach its food, raise the food and water bowls so that your dog does not have to flex its back or neck to eat and drink.

D. Transportation:
   1. When you are moving your dog, if your pet is in pain, you may wish to use a muzzle to prevent being bitten. Even a friendly dog may bite in reaction to pain. However, use a muzzle only if the dog is not having difficulty breathing and has not been vomiting. If at any time your dog has difficulty breathing, remove the muzzle. Also, do not use a muzzle if your dog has a flat face (e.g., a pug, boxer, Pekingese, English bulldog, etc.).
   2. **To transport a medium or large dog** that is unable to walk, obtain a plywood board or blanket to use as a stretcher. Slide your dog onto the board taking care to move your pet as little as possible. (Improper movement could cause severe damage, depending upon the dog's condition.) Place the plywood board with your dog on it into your vehicle. If the board will not fit, slide your dog off of the board and onto the seat with as little movement of your pet as possible. Unless your dog is overheated, pack blankets around your

104

dog to keep the pet warm. Also, unless your dog is overheated, place one or two 2-liter soda bottles filled with warm water (not hot water) against your dog. If you are concerned that your dog may slide off the seat onto the floor, pack the floor area with a pillow or blankets.

3.   **To transport a small dog** that is unable to walk, obtain a pet carrier that has a removable top. If a pet carrier is not available, use a corrugated cardboard box of an appropriate size. A carrier or box that opens at the top rather than the side is preferable because your dog can be put in and taken out without pushing or pulling. Slide your hands under your dog to lift. Take care to support your dog's entire body as you lift and place your dog into the carrier. Unless your dog is overheated, pack blankets around your dog to keep the pet warm. Also, unless your dog is overheated, place a 2-liter soda bottle filled with warm water (not hot water) against your dog. If you are concerned that your dog may slide off the seat onto the floor, pack the floor area with a pillow or blankets.

FLEAS AND TICKS

Fleas and ticks pose a substantial risk for the aging dog because older dogs tend to be physically weaker and more susceptible to illness. Fleas and ticks not only cause blood loss (sometimes resulting in anemia and death) but may also transmit diseases. A severe flea infestation may be extremely difficult to treat effectively, both in terms of your pet and your home. And an older dog may have more difficulty tolerating treatments necessary to get rid of the problem. Prevention and early treatment are essential in keeping the situation from developing into a major problem.

There are many flea products on the market, and you should ask your veterinarian which one will be best for your pet. Depending upon your dog's particular sensitivities, certain products may be much safer than others, and you should allow your veterinarian to make that determination.

Typically, when a dog has fleas, the dog will scratch itself; but not all dogs with fleas scratch themselves. A dog may show no obvious signs until weakness or disease appears. Therefore, it is important for you to check for fleas regularly by looking carefully at your dog's coat. Fleas are small, dark insects that jump or crawl through the dog's hair. Even if you cannot see the fleas, you may see flea droppings, which appear as black specks throughout the dog's hair coat. These black specks are actually the fleas' waste products.

Ticks can spread diseases, such as Rocky Mountain spotted fever, Ehrlechia and Lyme disease, and can also cause a condition called tick paralysis. Ticks are eight-legged parasites that are flat and sometimes have a hard, shiny covering. When they feed on a dog, they become enlarged and soft, and they can be mistaken for a mole on the dog's skin. Ticks often prefer to live on or near the dog's head and neck, but they may be found in any location. When a tick attaches itself, it embeds its mouth parts only. When you remove a tick, it is not possible for the head to get left behind in the dog's skin because the tick's head is not embedded. If the area of the tick bite becomes infected, it is generally from bacteria transmitted from the bite.

Whenever you are using flea products either as prevention or treatment for fleas or ticks, it is important to read all instructions thoroughly. Products that are used improperly or used in the wrong

106

combination can be harmful to your dog. Older dogs that are debilitated may be extremely sensitive to flea products, so consult your veterinarian before using any product. If your dog has an adverse reaction to any type of flea treatment, discontinue the treatment and contact a veterinarian immediately. The following instructions will help make your dog comfortable if fleas or ticks are a problem.

How to Improve Comfort

A. Consult your veterinarian if you suspect a problem with fleas or ticks. A number of external parasite-control protocols can be prescribed.

B. All flea products that you use on your dog should be labeled for use on dogs. These products should be used only as directed.

C. Examine your dog every time the pet comes into the house from outside, or at least once daily, for the presence of fleas or ticks.

D. Begin flea treatments as soon as you are aware of a flea problem. The longer you wait, the more difficult it will be to get rid of the fleas.

E. If you witness any unusual reactions to any flea treatments (e.g., drooling lasting longer than 20 minutes, tremors, seizures, respiratory difficulty, etc.), discontinue the treatments immediately, and contact your veterinarian.

F. Your dog and your home should be treated at the same time. Vacuum your home thoroughly, and then discard the vacuum cleaner bag. Wash your dog's bedding regularly. Using hand-held premises spray, treat all corners, baseboards, rugs, closets and cracks. Follow the instructions as directed on the product label. You may also use foggers strategically through the house in each closed room. Foggers will not penetrate through doorways or down hallways. Follow the instructions on the label.

G. Check environmental treatment inside the house two weeks after treatment by placing a pan of warm water on the floor before bedtime. Fleas are attracted to warmth and moisture, and if there are any remaining in your house, you should find some in the pan the next day. If you find that you have not eliminated the infestation, consult your veterinarian to discuss additional options.

H. Treat the yard with a yard and kennel spray as directed on the product label. Keep outside rest areas clean and dry.

I. To remove a tick, apply a flea and tick spray for dogs directly on the tick, and wait one minute. Then, using tweezers or wearing disposable gloves, apply constant pull while grasping the tick's body. The tick should release. Avoid touching the tick with your bare hands. Do not try to burn the tick or apply any other type of chemical to the tick. If flea or tick spray is not available, simply pull with constant pressure until the tick releases.

J. Dispose of the tick carefully. Make sure it is dead by spraying it with tick spray, or dispose of it by flushing it down the toilet.

K. Apply antibiotic ointment to the area where the tick was removed.

L. If any unusual symptoms develop after the removal of a tick, contact your veterinarian.

HEARING LOSS

Some hearing loss is almost universal in older dogs. It may be due to nerve degeneration or to the loss of sensory hairs in the middle ear. The loss of hearing is usually gradual, which gives the dog time to adjust to the change. Unhealthy ears may contribute to the deafness accompanying old age. Infections can cause swelling of the ear canal and thereby impede sound from entering the inner ear. Tumors or polyps in the ear may similarly interfere with hearing. The most common signs of deafness in a dog include: (1) the dog fails to respond to verbal commands, (2) the dog is difficult to awaken by verbal command, and (3) the dog is easily startled when approached, especially when approached from behind.

If the diminished hearing is due to infections or swellings, treatment will aid in improving hearing. A combination of antibiotic, anti-inflammatory, and surgery may be recommended. Signs that a dog may have unhealthy ears include shaking the head, scratching the ears, rubbing the ears on the floor, and crying when the ears are touched.

There are several ways to diagnose a hearing problem, and several ways to help your dog cope with deafness. See the outline below.

How to Improve Comfort

A. If you suspect that your dog may be losing its hearing, contact your veterinarian.

B. If there is visible debris in the ear, use an ear cleanser to clean the ears, or get veterinary help as soon as possible.

C. Teach your dog to recognize hand signals.

D. Keep your dog within safe boundaries (e.g., within a fenced yard), and do not allow your dog to roam.

E. When approaching from behind, create vibration (e.g., walk heavily) so the dog can feel you coming.

HEART DISEASE

Heart disease is a common occurrence in dogs. Heart disease may be a result of a birth defect, heartworm disease, infection, heart muscle disease, valve disease, cancer or aging. Regardless of the cause, the condition may be highly debilitating; however, many dogs have heart changes that they can live with comfortably. Recognizing symptoms early and getting help as soon as possible will increase your dog's comfort level and lengthen your dog's lifespan.

For all causes of heart disease, the range of symptoms is virtually identical. Dogs afflicted with heart disease will generally experience a chronic, nonproductive cough. Symptoms often include exercise intolerance, loss of appetite, abdominal distension and breathing difficulty. Eventually, as the condition progresses your dog may experience significant weakness or may even collapse.

Diagnosis of heart disease is usually made during a physical examination. Tests to confirm and to determine the cause of heart disease include X-rays or radiographs. (Radiography is a noninvasive way to look inside a dog to evaluate the size, shape, and position of the heart. It can also uncover the presence of fluids in the lungs or around the heart.)

Another test your veterinarian may use to diagnose heart disease is an electrocardiogram (also called an ECG or an EKG). The ECG is a noninvasive test that measures electrical activity in the heart. It is used to identify abnormalities in the heart's electrical activity or rhythm that can disrupt the heart's proper functioning. (An abnormal heart rhythm is called an arrhythmia.) An ECG can also confirm heart enlargement and provide information on the seriousness of a heart condition. Some changes in the ECG may also be suggestive of electrolyte imbalances or fluid around the heart.

A third commonly used heart test that is noninvasive is called an echocardiogram. The echocardiograph is an ultrasound of the heart that provides information on the size and efficiency of the heart as well as the functioning of the valves. It can also indicate the presence of fluid around the heart.

To properly diagnosis and treat heart disease, a veterinarian must perform certain blood tests to make sure your dog's other organs have not been affected by any changes in its heart and to make sure that your dog can take certain medicines without substantial risk of complications. Blood tests enable the veterinarian to prescribe the best type of medicine to control the problem. Treatment of heart disease is aimed toward improving the quality of life and lengthening your dog's lifespan.

The most common problem that affects the hearts of dogs is disease of the heart valves, especially the mitral valve which is located on the left side of the heart. One of these diseases, called endocardiosis, is characterized by a thickening of the heart valves that can cause the valves to leak. Although some breeds are more susceptible to valve disease than others, most dogs over the age of sixteen are afflicted with mitral valve problems. Some King Charles spaniels are afflicted at an especially early age; many of these dogs have valve problems by the age of two or three.

Heart valve disease is a condition that is usually detected by a veterinarian hearing a heart murmur during a routine checkup prior to the development of symptoms. Valve disease is usually slowly progressive. Early detection can enable the veterinarian to track the disease process and prescribe appropriate medications. The symptoms of the disease, like other heart problems, may include a chronic, nonproductive cough, exercise intolerance, weakness, loss of appetite, difficulty breathing, abdominal distension, and/or collapse. Blood tests, X-rays, an ECG, and an echocardiogram can confirm how advanced the disease process has become. Medicines help slow the progression of the disease by lowering the resistance the heart has to pump against. These medications usually help improve a dog's quality of life and extend its lifespan.

Infection on the heart valves, also known as endocarditis, is another condition that can affect dogs. Infection on the valves usually originates from another source in the body, such as infection in the mouth, urinary tract or lungs, and then migrates to the heart. Diagnosis of heart valve infection is through the usual heart tests. Infection can be treated with long-term antibiotics, and the symptoms of heart disease caused by the infection should receive appropriate therapy according to your dog's test results.

There are several types of heart muscle disease that can affect older dogs. The two most common are dilated cardiomyopathy (in which the heart muscle becomes flaccid, enlarged and inefficient) and cardiac hypertrophy (in which the heart muscle becomes thickened and inefficient). Dilated cardiomyopathy is second to valve disease as the most common heart ailment in older dogs. It commonly occurs in dogs between 4 to 10 years of age. It is a disease that affects larger, purebred breed dogs at a higher rate than mixed breed dogs. Breeds commonly affected include Scottish deerhounds, Doberman pinschers, Irish wolfhounds, Great Danes, boxers, Saint Bernards, Afghans, Newfoundlands and Old English sheepdogs. Medium size and smaller breed dogs are at lesser risk than larger dogs, except for the English and American cocker spaniels. Also, male dogs are almost twice as likely as female dogs to develop cardiomyopathy.

The symptoms of cardiomyopathy mirror those of other heart diseases and include a chronic, nonproductive cough, exercise intolerance, weakness, loss of appetite, difficulty breathing, abdominal distension and/or collapse. Diagnostic aids to determine the presence of cardiomyopathy include physical examination, blood tests, ECG's, X-rays, and echocardiograms. Medicines can be prescribed to help make the heart muscle a more efficient pump and to lower its work load.

Abnormal heart rhythms (called "arrhythmias") occur more commonly in older dogs. There are many types of arrhythmias ranging from abnormally high or abnormally low heart rates to fibrillation and flutter. (Fibrillation and flutter involve rapid, irregular beats of the heart muscle. Its seriousness depends on the part of the heart involved.) Atrioventricular block is another type of abnormal beat. It is characterized by a failure of the heart chambers to coordinate beats. Diagnosis is through the usual heart tests described earlier, but the ECG appears to be the most important aid. Medicines can be prescribed to help regulate the irregular heartbeats.

Regular veterinary examinations will help uncover heart disease early so that your dog can receive proper treatment to live a more comfortable, longer life. Most medicines prescribed act to lower blood pressure, remove extra fluids, change the heart rhythm, and make the heart contract more forcefully. Your veterinarian can explain the seriousness of the problem and help teach you CPR if the heart condition warrants.

How to Improve Comfort for a Dog with Heart Disease

A. Restrict activity until your dog can be checked by a veterinarian.

B. Repeat examinations may be necessary to determine the need to change any treatment to prolong your dog's life and provide comfort.

C. If your dog is having difficulty breathing, plan the handling of the dog to minimize excitement. Never hold the dog tightly.

D. Keep the dog in an upright position (i.e., belly down). Never lay the dog on its back or side because those positions make breathing more difficult by putting extra pressure on the chest.

E. Make sure you understand all instructions, the uses, and side effects of medications prescribed.

F. Give all medications on time according to the label.

G. Fresh water should always be available. Never withhold water from an older dog unless it is vomiting or unless you are advised to do so by your veterinarian.

H. Increase access to water by placing several water bowls throughout the house and where the dog lies.

I. Consider feeding your dog a prescription food that is low in sodium.

J. Avoid feeding your dog salty foods, such as commercial dog biscuits and other treats.

K. Avoid stressing any pet that has a chronic disease.

L. If your dog is weak, help your dog get outside to go to the bathroom at least four times per day.

M. Report any medication side effects to your veterinarian.

N. Learn CPR. See pages 180-181.

O. Report any changes in your dog's behavior or health to a veterinarian.

HYPOTHYROIDISM
(THYROID DEFICIENCY)

Hypothyroidism is a disease in which the dog's thyroid gland does not produce enough thyroid hormone. It is the most common hormonal disorder in dogs, affecting approximately 1 out of 500 dogs. The disease usually affects dogs that are over 4 years of age. Large breed dogs are at high risk, especially golden retrievers, Doberman pinschers, Irish setters, Airedale terriers, Great Danes and Old English sheepdogs. Some smaller breeds are also prone to hypothyroidism, such as miniature schnauzers, dachshunds, and cocker spaniels. The lack of thyroid hormone causes a variety of symptoms, but the most noticeable include loss of hair, weight gain and lack of activity. Other symptoms may include a change in the pigmentation of the dog's skin or shivering due to difficulty in maintaining the appropriate body temperature. Some dogs with hypothyroidism will appear to have a saddened or frowning appearance due to the thickening of skin in the area of the face. The changes described above tend to be gradual in onset.

Diagnosis of hypothyroidism is usually accomplished through a simple blood test that measures the amount of thyroid hormone in the blood. Treatment for the condition consists of providing your dog with a synthetic thyroid hormone replacement. The medicine is usually given once a day. Because the thyroid gland is not functioning properly in dogs with hypothyroidism, treatment is administered for the remainder of the dog's life. Follow-up blood testing is necessary to ensure the dog is on the correct dose.

How to Improve Comfort

A. If you detect any symptoms of hypothyroidism (described above) see your veterinarian to give your dog a blood test.

B. Until the diagnosis is made, keep your dog from chilling by providing a soft, warm bed.

C. Use all medications as prescribed by your veterinarian. If you

114

do not understand the instructions on the medicine, contact your veterinarian. Do not deviate from the dosage or the time interval on the label.

D.   Do not give medicine by mouth if your dog is vomiting.

E.   Unless specifically directed by your veterinarian, do not mix medicine in your dog's food; your dog may refuse to eat or not get all of its medicine.

F.   Consider using a food that is lower in calories. Ask your veterinarian for recommendations.

G.   Have your dog's thyroid level checked regularly as recommended by your veterinarian.

INCONTINENCE (URINARY)

Urinary incontinence refers to the inability to control urinations at regular intervals. There are many different causes of urinary incontinence, ranging from bladder irritations and disease conditions to changes in hormones. In many cases, incontinence is not just a normal aging change. Often it signifies a more serious medical condition. Nerve degeneration or metabolic changes taking place in the internal organs, such as the kidneys, liver, and pancreas can result in increased urinations. Often medical treatment can help.

There are several signs of incontinence that you may observe. Your dog's hair surrounding its genitals may become stained with urine, or you may observe a puddle where your dog is, or was, lying. There are some less obvious signs you might note, if you are observant: Your dog may experience dribbling or leakage of urine either during sleep or when awake; your dog may have an increased volume or frequency of urinations; or your dog may have increased thirst and expel urine that looks like water. Report any signs that you observe to your veterinarian.

Bladder irritations can cause a dog to urinate without control. Usually the intervals between urinations become shorter and may result in accidents in the house. The quantity of urine is usually smaller because it is expelled more frequently. Other symptoms include straining, blood in the urine, and urgency. Causes of irritations include bladder infections, bladder crystals and/or stones. These changes can be observed in dogs of any age but become more common as dogs become older.

Obstruction may also cause incontinence. Bladder stones, tumors, and prostatic enlargement may partially obstruct the outflow of urine, causing the leakage of urine as pressure in the bladder increases. If the obstruction becomes a complete blockage, it is a life-threatening emergency, and your dog should be rushed to a veterinarian immediately.

Changes in hormones can also play a role in urinary incontinence. Older female spayed dogs may suffer from a condition called hormone-responsive incontinence, in which the dog starts to dribble urine, especially when resting. This condition responds well to estrogen therapy.

Excess cortisol hormone can cause symptoms of incontinence.

116

The increased cortisol levels with Cushing's disease (see pages 84-86) can cause an increased loss of fluids through the kidneys. Also a decrease or absence of insulin production, resulting in diabetes, will cause the loss of sugar in the urine and result in increased urine production. In both conditions, it is difficult for the bladder to store the increased volume, which can result in loss of urinary control; you may observe your dog leaking urine when asleep, or you may notice increased volumes of urine and/or a greater urge for your dog to go out more often. Increased thirst may also occur with Cushing's disease or diabetes. Medical and sometimes surgical treatment are recommended for these diseases.

Changes in organ function may also cause increased volume of urine. These changes are commonly seen with liver and kidney disease. Also, excess salt intake, imbalances in calcium, and certain medications (e.g., prednisone or furosemide) can cause increased volume of urine. When the cause of incontinence is a medication, the incontinence usually goes away when the dosage is decreased or when the medication is discontinued.

Unhealthy changes in the uterus can also result in increased urine production and incontinence. Infection of the uterus (pyometra) can occur for no apparent reason in a seemingly normal, healthy dog. The cause is generally hormonal, and prior to symptoms, there is no method of predicting when or whether it might occur. The unspayed, older female is at highest risk. Most female dogs over the age of five years have some uterus thickening, and when the uterus thickens, it is more susceptible to infection. If an infection occurs, the uterus can fill with pus, and the pressure from the infection can cause the uterus to burst, spilling infection into the abdomen. Also, an infection in the uterus can spread into the bloodstream and can be fatal.

One symptom of a uterus infection is increased thirst, which sometimes appears prior to the development of other symptoms. General signs of illness, such as loss of appetite and decreased energy may accompany the presence of a cloudy discharge from the vulvar area. Note, however, that a discharge is not always present with an infection of the uterus. Also, in some cases, the abdomen becomes tense or enlarged. Treatment for a uterine infection includes getting the dog stabilized and then surgically removing the uterus. Other forms of treatment with antibiotics and hormones have proved unsuccessful.

Nerve injury, or more commonly nerve degeneration, can also be a cause of incontinence. Degenerative myelopathy is a nerve disorder that affects large breed dogs, most commonly German shepherds. The symptoms include weakness and loss of coordination in the rear legs. Often the toes of the hind legs will knuckle under and scrape on the ground. Urinary incontinence and loss of bowel control are common symptoms. Unfortunately there is no treatment for this disorder; it usually gets progressively worse over time.

Good hygiene (i.e., promptly washing away any urine that gets onto the dog's coat and maintaining clean, dry bedding) is one of the most important treatments to help care for your dog until the cause of the incontinence can be determined. Urine can cause severe inflammation of the skin, referred to as urine scald. This condition is painful and can result in infection. Also, it hastens the development of decubital ulcers (pressure sores) on dogs that have difficulty getting up.

How to Improve Comfort

A. When you suspect that your dog has become incontinent, contact your veterinarian for help. In most cases, medical intervention will treat the problem.

B. Measure the amount of water your dog drinks. If the amount exceeds one cup per day for every 7 pounds of the dog's body weight (e.g., 5 cups per day for a 35 pound dog), under moderate environmental conditions, report this to your veterinarian.

C. Never restrict water from a dog with excess thirst.

D. Keep the dog clean around the genitals. At least four times daily, use baby wipes or mild soap and water, and rinse well.

E. Apply antibiotic ointment (e.g., Polysporin®) to any sore areas.

F. Lightly apply corn starch powder to area if no breathing difficulty exists.

G. Apply a diaper if necessary. (See pages 177-178.)
    1. Place diaper between dog's legs.
    2. Insert tail through hole.
    3. Pull adhesive tabs up then reinforce them with masking tape. You may need to stick a small portion of tape to the hair to keep the diaper on.
    4. Change the diaper as needed.

INFECTIONS AND FEVER

Infections and fever are unpredictable when left unattended. Many mild infections and fevers may resolve on their own; however, some can be overwhelming and cause long-term complications or death. The likelihood of a poor outcome is greater with an older pet whose immune system may be compromised. Also, underlying diseases that are most prevalent in older dogs, such as diabetes or Cushing's disease, make the older dog more predisposed to infections. And decayed teeth, also generally associated with age, make dogs prone to infections because germs in the mouth can easily enter the bloodstream when the gums are unhealthy. Underlying disease may also make infections difficult to overcome because the immune system can become overwhelmed. Common infections seen in aging dogs include mouth infections, urinary tract infections, infectious bronchitis, sinus infections and skin infections.

Signs of infections include, but are not limited to, loss of appetite, weakness, lethargy, vomiting, diarrhea, fever, pain or swelling over an area, and/or disorientation. Your dog might not show any outward signs until the infection becomes advanced. For example, if your dog has decaying teeth with a low-grade infection in its mouth, the infection might not be apparent until it has spread through the blood to the heart valves and kidneys.

Veterinarians typically diagnose infections through physical examinations, blood tests, cultures, and response to treatments. Other testing, such as X-rays and ultrasound, may be required to pinpoint the source of infection. Regardless of the cause of the infection, early diagnosis and treatment will hasten recovery. These following guidelines will improve the comfort of a pet suffering from an infection.

How to Improve Comfort

A. When you suspect that your dog has an infection, contact your veterinarian immediately; antibiotics may be necessary.

B. If the dog's condition, while on medication, does not improve, or if it worsens, again contact your veterinarian. The veterinarian may need to change medications or may decide to perform more tests to better identify the problem.

C. Use all medications as prescribed by your veterinarian.

D. Do not deviate from the dosage or the time interval on the label.

E. Use all antibiotics until they are gone, unless directed otherwise. Sporadic use of antibiotics can cause bacteria to become resistant to treatment.

F. Increased nutritional intake will often hasten recovery. Consider giving your pet a dog multivitamin. Consult with your veterinarian about increasing food intake and vitamins.

G. Take your dog's temperature daily to monitor progress. Normal temperature should be between 101 and 103 degrees Fahrenheit.

INNER EAR OR VESTIBULAR DISEASE

The vestibular system helps control balance, posture and head position. The vestibular system includes the inner ear, plus related nerves and parts of the brainstem and cerebellum. Any injury, infection, tumor or inflammation in the vestibular system can cause stroke-like symptoms.

Signs of vestibular disease include a head tilt, disorientation, confusion, stumbling, loss of balance, walking in circles, and involuntary eye movement (side-to-side). In some cases, loss of appetite, nausea and vomiting may occur.

A common cause of vestibular disease in dogs is idiopathic vestibular syndrome (often referred to as geriatric vestibular syndrome when it occurs in older dogs). This condition affects mostly older dogs, at an average age of twelve or thirteen years, and it affects males and females in equal proportions. The syndrome comes on quickly, sometimes within two hours. Many times vestibular disease is mistaken for a stroke. It may be more severe during the first few days, causing your dog to fall or rendering your dog unable to walk. Head tilt, disorientation, confusion, stumbling, loss of balance, walking in circles, and involuntary eye movement may occur. This condition affects the appetite and causes nausea in approximately one-third of the dogs inflicted. The symptoms usually last one to three weeks but can extend up to six weeks. The condition improves with time. Recovery from idiopathic vestibular syndrome is usually excellent.

Because there is no specific test for this condition, it is diagnosed based on its symptoms, physical examination, and by ruling out other causes. The cause of this condition is unknown, and therefore treatment is aimed at keeping your dog comfortable by treating the signs and providing good nursing care.

Nursing care consists of keeping your dog nourished, preventing dehydration, and maintaining good hygiene. Especially during the first few days, your dog may have difficulty taking care of itself because of dizziness. If your dog is not vomiting, you may need to move food and water near your dog to provide better access. In

121

some cases, you may have to offer food and water by hand six to eight times per day. It is important to help your dog get up and down to help preserve muscle strength, to improve circulation, and to provide ample opportunity for your dog to go outside to go to the bathroom.

Proper footing is extremely important for dogs that have difficulty getting up and down. Slippery floors are hazardous because they do not provide the necessary traction for your dog, and slipping can result in injury. Provide your dog with a good surface consisting of nonskid throw rugs, bath mats or industrial rubber mats. Towels and blankets are soft but too slippery to be useful.

To lift and move a medium sized to large dog that does not have the strength to help, put one arm under the dog's stomach (below the ribs) and the other hand under the dog's neck (with the dog's neck in the corner formed by your elbow). When lifting your dog, bend your knees and lift with equal pressure on both arms. If your strength does not permit you to lift your dog, tuck a blanket under your dog or roll your dog onto a blanket and then transport your dog by pulling on the blanket, or have someone help as the two of you lift opposite corners of the blanket.

To help your dog rise from a sitting or lying position, place a towel under the dog's abdomen, and place another towel between the front legs. Lift the front towel first using equal pressure on both ends of that towel. Once the front end is almost up, start to lift the back towel. If available, cloth log carriers with handles can be substituted for the towels to help support your dog. Note that your dog is depending upon you for its balance, and be careful not to let your dog stumble and hit its nose on the ground.

Your dog should be kept clean and dry to prevent complications, such as pressure sores and skin infections. Your dog should be kept combed and brushed daily in order to remove dirt and dying hair from its coat. This daily attention also will increase circulation.

Toenails should be trimmed as often as necessary; a debilitated dog has decreased activity and therefore may not wear down its nails to the extent that a younger dog typically does. Long nails will cause your dog to stand improperly on its feet, creating unnatural stress on bones and ligaments, which can cause pain or aggravate arthritis. Problems with toenails will also cause an already dizzy dog even more difficulty maintaining balance and walking.

With certain breeds, caring for a debilitated dog may be easier if its hair coat is kept short. At the very least, be sure to keep the hair

122

trimmed around the eyes, ears, mouth, and feet. Hair should also be trimmed away from the rectum and genitals to provide better hygiene and to facilitate ease of cleaning those areas.

The process of bathing may become more complicated when your dog has vestibular disease because standing for a bath may be difficult. In addition to regular baths, if your dog becomes soiled with urine or feces, bathe the dog immediately. Use baby wipes or mild soap and water, and then rinse well and dry. Apply triple antibiotic ointment to any sore areas. Lightly apply corn starch powder to the genital area, provided that your dog does not have difficulty breathing. Repeat this cleaning process for your dog's genital area as many times per day as necessary.

A walk-in shower with a spray nozzle is the most convenient method of bathing larger breed dogs. A bath towel or mat may be placed in the bottom of the shower or tub to provide traction for your dog to prevent slipping. During warmer weather, a dog can be bathed outside using a hose hook-up to a faucet that provides warm water (e.g., a sink as opposed to an outside gardening faucet). Never bathe a dog in cold water because cold water can cause hypothermia and muscle soreness. If a whole body bath is not required, wash only the soiled area. Be sure to keep urine and stool off the coat to prevent infection and sores from developing.

Proper bedding improves your dog's comfort during the recovery process. The most important feature of a good bed is cleanliness. Materials that are easy to wash are desirable. Examples of good bedding include folded comforters, commercial stuffed beds with removable, waterproof covers, or rubber mats covered with a blanket or towels. Foam-like materials should be avoided unless a waterproof covering is available. Waterbeds, though easy to clean, need to be carefully monitored for proper temperature. Make sure that the bed you provide is large enough to allow your dog to stretch out and lie flat. Proper thickness depends upon the type of material used, but the bedding should be thick enough to provide soft padding and insulation from the floor. Soft padding is important to prevent pressure sores from developing.

A variety of aids can be used if the dog is incontinent and leaks urine while in bed. A diaper may be used as described on pages 177-178. Or an absorbable pad may be placed under your dog to remove any wetness or moisture from the dog's skin. Washing the bedding may be facilitated by having spare bedding available, especially if frequent soiling occurs. Bedding may also be protected by placing a layer of plastic (e.g., plastic trash bags), or similar waterproof material, over the bedding and then placing a towel over the plastic. Note, however, that use of plastic can make the bed slip and slide. A waterproof bed liner that is not slippery would be ideal. When bedding does get soiled, it should be washed immediately. Urine and stool saturated bedding promotes infection and pressure sores if the dog spends much time in bed.

A dog's bed should be situated in a draft-free, dry, well-ventilated area. This should be a supervised area of the house so that you can interact with your dog and observe your dog's behavior and habits. Try to avoid dark, damp basements. Your dog's food and water should be near the bed so that there is easy access.

Remember, a dog with vestibular syndrome is depending upon you for temporary help until the condition runs its course. The nursing care may be more rigorous during the first week, but the rewards are great because the prognosis is excellent.

How to Improve Comfort

A. If your dog is disoriented or appears to have a loss of balance or coordination, block off stairways, and restrict the pet's activity.

B. Seek veterinary care as soon as possible.

C. If your dog shows no sign of nausea, offer food and water by hand feeding.

D. Carry or help your dog outside to go to the bathroom four times per day.

E. Provide good bedding.
    1. Keep all bedding clean.
    2. Provide a bed large enough for your dog to lie flat.
    3. Locate the bed in a draft-free, dry, well-ventilated environment.
    4. Locate the bed where your dog can be closely monitored.

F. Keep food and water in close proximity.

G. Maintain your dog's grooming.
    1. Comb or brush your dog daily.
    2. Keep your dog's toenails trimmed.
    3. Trim hair around tail area and genitals for easier hygiene.

H. Keep your dog clean.
    1. Never bathe your dog in cold water.
    2. Rinse well of soap; then dry your dog well.

3. Partial baths can be used to wash small soiled areas. Keep your dog clean around the genitals at least four times daily with baby wipes or mild soap and water. Rinse well.
4. Apply triple antibiotic ointment to any sore areas.
5. Lightly apply corn starch powder to area if no breathing difficulty exists.

I. Contact your veterinarian regarding any complications.

INTESTINAL PARASITES

Intestinal parasites, which include worms and protozoa, can cause serious illness if untreated. Parasites place additional stress on an aging dog's health. Most infestations are mild at first but then become serious as time progresses. If parasites are left untreated, fatal anemia, from chronic blood loss, and life-threatening malnutrition can develop. The most common parasites in dogs include roundworms, tapeworms, hookworms and whipworms. Protozoa infestations include coccidia and giardia. Some of these infections can be spread to people.

The signs of intestinal parasites may include weight loss, diarrhea or soft stools, bloody stools, mucous in the stool, listlessness, vomiting, pot-bellied appearance, and/or dull hair coat. However, signs might not be apparent, and the condition can go undetected. Therefore, you should have your dog's stool sample checked under the microscope by a veterinarian at least twice per year. By checking a stool with a microscope, a veterinarian can detect worm eggs and protozoa. If any parasites are present, your veterinarian can prescribe the proper medication.

Prevention, Detection and Treatment

A. Clean your yard of stools at least once per day.

B. Practice good flea control. Fleas spread one type of tapeworm.

C. Never feed a dog raw meat.

D. Provide clean, fresh water for your outdoor dog because outside water may contain infectious protozoa or bacteria.

E. Have a stool specimen examined by a veterinarian at least twice per year.

F. If you see any worms in the stool, contact your veterinarian.

G. Avoid over-the-counter worm medications; they may not be the proper choice for your pet's illness.

H. Use worm medications as directed.

KIDNEY DISEASE

A variety of kidney diseases plague dogs; however, the most common kidney problem seen in aging dogs is chronic renal failure. The average age at which a dog is typically diagnosed with chronic renal disease is approximately seven years. One to two percent of dogs between the ages of seven and ten suffer from this disease. While some breeds may be particularly susceptible to developing kidney disorders (e.g., golden retrievers, Doberman pinschers, Lhasa apsos, Shih Tzus, Norwegian elkhounds, cocker spaniels, Samoyeds, standard poodles, and soft-coated wheaten terriers), the problem is experienced by all breeds of dogs.

Chronic renal disease is a progressive condition in which the kidneys lose their function at a slow rate. There are many causes of chronic renal failure, ranging from infection, inflammation, and cancer, to genetic and normal aging change. Even if the cause of the condition is remedied, the kidney function may continue to decline because typically 50-75% of the kidney function is lost before signs of kidney failure become apparent.

As a dog ages, its kidney weight and size decrease. Because of the reduced size and function of the aging kidneys, the kidneys may become more sensitive to changes and stresses. The severity of symptoms of chronic renal failure depend on the age of the dog, any other disease processes, the cause of the condition, the severity, and the duration of the condition.

When the kidneys fail, there is a buildup of poisons in the blood (called azotemia or uremia). Blood pressure increases, electrolytes (such as phosphorus and potassium) become imbalanced, and anemia occurs. Because of these abnormalities, many additional problems occur in other areas of the body. The early signs of chronic renal failure include increased thirst, decreased appetite, weakness and depression. Dogs may begin to drink excessive amounts of water and need to go outside more often. This may first become evident by dogs having accidents in the house, especially at night. Over time, weight loss may occur. The dog may lose its appetite, become nauseated, vomit, and/or develop diarrhea. Oral ulcers may also develop and affect appetite. Increased blood pressure may have adverse affects on vision, possibly by causing detached retinas or glaucoma. Blindness can result. Increased blood pressure can also put an additional burden on the heart. The buildup of poisons may also affect the nervous system by causing tremors, disorientation, confusion, loss of balance, and seizures. The longer the condition remains untreated, the more likely it is that you will begin to observe some of these signs.

Diagnosis of chronic renal failure is usually based on blood tests. Urine tests, cultures, ultrasound, kidney biopsy, and X-rays are also helpful in determining the origin of the problem.

Depending upon your dog's symptoms, a veterinarian's treatment for the problems that result from chronic renal failure may include some of the following: If the dog is dehydrated, your veterinarian may recommend intravenous fluids or subcutaneous fluids (i.e., fluids under the skin). Antacids, such as cimetidine (Tagamet®) or Pepsid®, may be used to help control stomach acid buildup. Medications such as metaclopromide or Reglan® may help control nausea and loss of appetite. Medicines such as some antibiotics and heart drugs may need to have their dosages adjusted to accommodate for kidney changes in drug metabolism. Certain drugs for other ailments must be closely monitored for side effects that may hinder appetite. Vitamin B and iron should be supplemented to enhance appetite and to help with anemia. Appetite may be stimulated by the administration of anabolic steroids. The drug Epogen® can be given to help anemia. Increased phosphorus levels may be controlled by giving an antacid that binds phosphorus or by administering calcitriol. Potassium can be supplemented if needed. Sodium bicarbonate may be prescribed to counter the effects of a condition called acidosis. Your veterinarian may recommend changes to your pet's diet as the disease progresses.

How to Improve Comfort

A. Report any sign of kidney failure to your veterinarian. Initial signs may include increased thirst, increased frequency of urination, wetting in the house, weakness, depression, confusion, vomiting or diarrhea.

B. Modify the dog's diet and feeding.

    1. Ask your veterinarian for recommendations.

    2. Make any change in diet gradually over a period of one to two weeks.

    3. If necessary, add flavor enhancers (such as bouillon, garlic,

and/or clam juice) to your dog's food to increase palatability.

4. Feed your dog several small meals daily.

5. Warm your dog's food to enhance the smell.

C. Provide a good vitamin supplement that contains vitamin B and iron. Ask your veterinarian.

D. Provide access to several bowls of fresh water.

E. Avoid stress (e.g., long trips, hot weather, any extreme conditions).

F. Report any unusual signs to your doctor so that appropriate support medication can be prescribed as needed.

LUMPS AND BUMPS

An aging dog is more prone to developing lumps, bumps or skin masses. These changes in and on your dog's body may be due to causes that range from minor insect bites to life-threatening cancers. Other causes include swollen lymph nodes, blocked anal glands, blocked salivary glands, and a variety of different types of cysts. Although most lumps and bumps commonly occur on, in, or under the skin, there are some that can occur internally, such as tumors of the spleen, liver, and bowels.

Dogs should be checked at least once every week for the development of lumps and bumps. This is best accomplished by starting at the dog's nose and working your way back to the tail. By running your hands slowly over the dog's entire body, you will be able to identify any unusual changes. Don't forget to check around the rectum and between the toes and on the pads of the feet. If any lumps/bumps are found, you should make note whether they are on the skin surface, in the skin, or under the skin. You should also record the size and location. All lumps and bumps should be checked by a veterinarian to determine their origin and nature. A previously diagnosed lump should be rechecked if the growth changes in size, shape or color because it is possible for a benign lump to turn into a malignant growth.

To diagnose the origin and nature of a suspicious lump, a veterinarian may recommend a fine needle aspirate (a technique in which a needle is inserted into the lump, and cells are removed for examination under a microscope), an impression smear (a technique whereby cells are gathered by touching a slide to the mass; then the cells are examined under a microscope), or perhaps removal and biopsy of the lump.

Skin masses may be either benign or malignant. A malignant skin bump has the potential to get progressively worse by growing in size, invading surrounding areas, or spreading to different sites in the body (metastasis). A benign skin growth, unlike a malignancy, does not spread or invade the body. The only definite way to determine whether a bump is malignant or benign is to have it tested through a biopsy or fine needle aspirate.

Common skin tumors in older dogs include basal cell tumors, cutaneous lymphoma, mast cell tumors, melanomas, papillomas, perianal gland tumors, sebaceous gland tumors, and squamous cell carcinoma. Treatment of these problem tumors usually includes surgical removal, sometimes followed by chemotherapy or radiation treatments.

How to Improve Comfort

A. Check your dog weekly for any skin bumps by running your hand over your dog's body from nose to tail.
B. Look in the mouth and under the tail for lumps.
C. If any bumps break open, gently wash the area using antiseptic soap, and then apply antibiotic ointment to the area, and contact your veterinarian.
D. Contact your veterinarian if you detect any change in size, shape, or color of any previously discovered growth.

OSTEOPOROSIS

There are two types of osteoporosis in dogs: one resulting from normal aging, and the other caused by disease processes. Osteoporosis that is caused by aging is less significant in dogs than it is in people. Osteoporosis from aging rarely makes a dog susceptible to fractures, though it does slow healing of fractures. When osteoporosis is caused by disease processes, it may have a more profound effect on bones, and even ligaments, and these dogs may be more prone to fractures. Diseases associated with osteoporosis include hyperparathyroidism, renal failure, Cushing's disease, diabetes, and hyperthyroidism.

Because of the effect that many diseases have on bone strength, any changes in your dog's health should be investigated to help prevent the weakening of bones, as well as to prevent any other unwanted side effects from the disease process. If your veterinarian determines that your dog is at risk for a fracture, pay careful attention to any changes in the dog's movements. In particular, be aware that a dog usually will not bear weight on a fractured leg. A fractured limb may appear swollen, and typically it will not improve with time. Fractures of the ribs may be associated with difficult breathing as well as tenderness in the fractured area.

How to Improve Comfort for a Dog with Osteoporosis

A. If your dog has been diagnosed with a disease that can cause osteoporosis, follow specific treatment instructions closely to help prevent weak bones.

B. Avoid rough activities.

C. If a fracture or lameness does occur, seek veterinary help.

1. Because fractures are painful, you may wish to use a muzzle to prevent being bitten when you move your dog. However, use a muzzle only if your dog is not having difficulty breathing and has not been vomiting. If at any time your dog has difficulty breathing, remove the muzzle. Also, do not use a muzzle if your dog has a flat face (e.g., a pug,

132

boxer, English bulldog, etc.).

2. Keep your dog still. If necessary, wrap the pet in a towel or blanket to restrict its movements.

3. Keep any open wounds covered with gauze and secure with tape. If an open wound is bleeding profusely, apply pressure over that area.

4. Plan your transportation to the veterinarian carefully to minimize movement of your dog.

REPRODUCTIVE PROBLEMS – FEMALE

Many reproductive changes occur in aging female dogs, especially in those that are not altered (i.e., not spayed). While there are various types of reproductive diseases in female dogs, including various cancers, the most common problem is uterine infections. Infection of the uterus (called pyometras) can occur for no apparent reason in a seemingly healthy dog. The cause is generally hormonal, and prior to symptoms, there is no method of predicting when or whether it might occur. Infections of the uterus can be fatal. The unspayed, older female is at greatest risk. Most female dogs over the age of five have some thickening of the uterus, which can lead quickly to pyometras. When a dog's uterus ages, it thickens and can fill with a pus-like discharge which can lead to infection. Eventually, in the most serious cases, the uterus can burst, spilling bacteria into the abdomen or into the bloodstream. One symptom of a uterine infection is increased thirst, sometimes prior to the development of other signs. General signs of illness, such as loss of appetite and energy, may appear in conjunction with a cloudy discharge from the vulvar area. (Note: Discharge is not always present when there is a uterine infection.) The abdomen may or may not be tense or distended. Treatment for a uterine infection includes getting the dog stabilized and then surgically removing the uterus. Other forms of treatment (e.g., antibiotics and hormones) have proved unsuccessful. Diagnosis of reproductive diseases is usually through examinations, blood tests, X-rays, ultrasound, and biopsies.

Prevention and Comfort

A. The best prevention is to have your female dog spayed before any reproductive problems develop.

B. If any symptoms of reproductive disease appear (e.g., vulvar discharge), contact a veterinarian immediately. If your female dog has a uterine infection, the condition is a medical emergency; your dog may require an emergency spay before the uterus ruptures.

1. When transporting your dog, do not lift your dog by putting extra pressure on its abdomen; lifting in that manner may cause a damaged uterus to rupture.

2. To help prevent shock, place a 2-liter soda bottle filled with warm water (not hot water) next to your dog (as illustrated below).

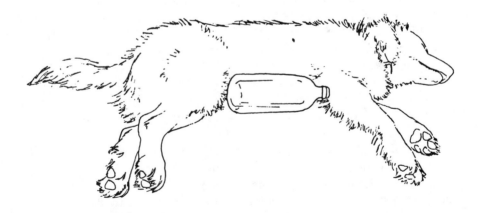

REPRODUCTIVE PROBLEMS
– MALE

Many reproductive changes occur in the male dog during the aging process. Problems more commonly encountered in dogs that are not altered (i.e., not neutered) include enlarged prostate glands, prostatic cancer, and testicular tumors.

As a male dog ages, the risk of prostatic problems increases if the dog has not been neutered. Dogs as young as four years of age may start developing problems. Dobermans and German shepherds have a particularly high incidence. When the prostate gland becomes enlarged due to the development of cysts, infection, or cancer, it causes a variety of complications. It can compress the rectum resulting in straining during bowel movements, and it can become so severe that constipation can develop. It may also put pressure on the urethra, causing difficulty urinating. Infection in the prostate gland may result in other signs of illness, such as fever, weakness, vomiting, diarrhea, urinary irritation, and discharge from the penis. The diagnosis of prostatic problems is usually made through a rectal examination, blood tests, x-rays, and ultrasound.

The usual treatment of choice for an enlarged prostate gland is castration. Castration quickly reduces the size of the gland, thereby providing relief from some of the symptoms. Castration is preferred over hormonal therapy if the dog is a good surgical candidate because hormones have serious side effects.

The prostate gland is also susceptible to cysts and infections. Cysts of the prostate gland may require special surgical removal or drainage. Infection in the prostate gland requires long-term antibiotic therapy for at least six weeks.

Older male dogs also have a higher incidence of cancer of the testicles. Testicular cancer is a common cancer in male dogs and is particularly common in German shepherds, Shetland sheepdogs, and Weimaraners. Dogs that have undescended testicles are at a significantly higher risk of developing tumors compared to normal dogs. Fortunately, most testicular tumors are benign. However, the small percentage that are malignant can spread to lymph nodes, the liver, and the lungs. With certain testicular tumors, excess estrogen (female hormone) is produced, and when that occurs, the dog can

136

develop breasts that produce milk, and the dog may also lose its hair, experience skin darkening, and possibly become anemic. Signs of testicular tumors include the above plus the development of any lumps or bumps on the testicles, and increased size of one or both testicles. The treatment of choice is neutering.

Prevention and Comfort

A. The best way to prevent prostatic problems and testicular cancer in a male dog is to have the dog neutered.

B. Contact a veterinarian if you observe your dog straining to defecate or urinate, or if you observe a discharge from the dog's penis, a lack of appetite, vomiting, or diarrhea.

C. Once every month, gently feel your dog's testicles for lumps, bumps or enlargements. Report any changes to your veterinarian.

D. Changes such as hair loss, breast development, milk production, and darkening of skin are warning signs and should be reported to a veterinarian.

SEIZURES

A seizure consists of involuntary convulsing that occurs because of abnormal electrical impulses traveling through the brain. Seizures are a common phenomenon in dogs. They can be caused by a number of problems that change the brain's function, including blood sugar imbalances (sometimes from diabetes), head trauma, various poisons, electrolyte imbalances, or a buildup of wastes in the dog's circulation (i.e., as a result of organ failure). In young dogs, seizures may be hereditary or congenital in nature. Breeds of dogs that are particularly susceptible to seizures include German shepherds, Irish setters, miniature poodles, Siberian huskies, beagles, cocker spaniels, Labrador retrievers, keeshonden and miniature schnauzers.

A seizure may present itself in a variety of ways. It may be generalized affecting the whole body, or it may be partial affecting only certain parts of the body, such as a single limb. The seizures may also start as partial or localized and then turn into a generalized event. The partial seizure may last up to thirty minutes, whereas a generalized one is usually less than five minutes. Seizures may be mild (petit mal) or severe (grand mal). A seizure that will not stop on its own is referred to as status epilepticus.

A seizure can present as twitching, confusion, rage, fear, jerking or stiffness, chewing, licking, running, turning, and/or circling. Some dogs will even go through a routine where they act as if they are biting at imaginary flies or chasing their tails. A dog may drool, urinate, defecate or sometimes vomit during a seizure. After a seizure, a dog may go through a recovery (postictal) phase where it may have side effects ranging from being depressed to being blind for several hours or several days.

A diagnosis is aimed at determining the cause of the seizure, through a neurologic examination, blood tests, urinalysis, X-rays, ultrasound, EEG (electroencephalogram), MRI, or CT scan. If a diagnosis cannot be determined, the dog is then said to have idiopathic (i.e., arising spontaneously from unknown cause) epilepsy. If a cause is determined, treatment should be directed toward correcting the underlying problem with the goal of decreasing the frequency, severity, and duration of the seizures, and decreasing the aftereffect of the seizures. In addition to treating the underlying cause, there are several medications specifically used to help control or prevent seizures. Some of the medications may cause drowsiness, but this drowsiness may eventually pass when the dog becomes accustomed to the medication. Contact your veterinarian regarding any side effects.

Seizures are frightening events to watch. Try to stay calm so that you are best able to tend to your dog's needs.

How to Improve Comfort

A. If a seizure is occurring, note the time on a clock or watch and measure the duration of the event.

B. If the seizure lasts more than 2 minutes, get veterinary help immediately; the condition may be life threatening.

C. Move any objects away from the dog if they could cause injury.

D. Block any stairways.

E. Never place your fingers in a dog's mouth during a seizure.

F. If the seizure stops and the dog appears lifeless, proceed with CPR. See pages 180-181.

G. If the seizure stops at home, even if your pet seems normal, consult your veterinarian as soon as possible.

H. If your dog has been diagnosed with seizures, record each time a seizure occurs.

I. Record any common events that tie the seizures together (e.g., noise, lights, trauma).

J. If your dog is taking medication for seizures and the seizures do not improve, again contact your veterinarian. You may need to change medications or the veterinarian may need to perform a blood test to determine whether the dose should be adjusted.

    1. Use all medications as prescribed by your veterinarian.

    2. Do not deviate from the dosage or the time interval on the label.

    3. Renew prescriptions on a timely basis. Do not run out of tablets or allow your dog to skip any doses.

SHAKING

Older dogs have a tendency to shiver or shake more often than younger dogs. There are many causes of shaking, including a chill, fear, weakness, poisons, potassium excess, calcium deficiency, low blood sugar, brain changes, and nerve changes. Perhaps the most common causes of shaking in older dogs are chills from a thyroid hormone deficiency or from disease processes that make it difficult for the dog to maintain its body temperature. Another cause is a condition called senile tremors, which affects older dogs and usually causes the rear legs to shake when the dog is standing, but subsides when the dog is lying down or active. The cause of this condition is unknown, although it does not appear to cause serious complications.

How to Improve Comfort

A.   If shaking or shivering occurs, contact a veterinarian to determine the cause.

B.   Provide your dog with extra warmth in the form of a blanket or warm water bottle.

C.   If your dog is underweight, provide a wholesome diet.

D.   Ask your veterinarian about adding a multivitamin to your dog's diet.

E.   Note any signs of illness (e.g., loss of appetite, weakness, tiredness, vomiting, or diarrhea).

SKIN CONDITIONS

Skin conditions and hair loss in the older dog can cause much discomfort and can be a warning sign of other more serious diseases. Compared to young dogs, older dogs are more affected by skin problems, especially metabolic diseases that cause hair loss. As the skin ages, it loses its oils, causing a dry coat. Also, the hair becomes thinner from the loss of follicles, and the skin loses some of its elasticity. Signs of skin conditions include excess shedding, missing hair, reddened skin, painful skin, and/or scratching. Other accompanying signs of illness, such as increased thirst, lethargy, panting, vomiting, diarrhea, and weight gain may signify a complicated skin condition.

Some diseases, such as hypothyroidism and Cushing's disease, usually cause hair loss in affected dogs. Hypothyroidism is a disease whereby the dog does not make enough thyroid hormone. The lack of thyroid hormone causes hair loss, tiredness, increased weight gain, and sometimes chills. Cushing's disease also causes hair loss and can be responsible for a number of other serious symptoms, including increased thirst and urinations, distension of the abdomen (barrel with legs appearance), panting, weight gain, and/or increased appetite. Cushing's disease is caused when the body makes too much cortisol or when an excess of cortisone therapy has been prescribed.

In people, allergies often cause sneezing, runny eyes, and wheezing, whereas in dogs, allergies usually cause itching and rashes, which can cause hair loss. Allergies in dogs can be caused by a number of irritants, including pollens, grasses, dusts, and molds, as well as any foods for which the dog might have a particular sensitivity. The degree of a dog's discomfort from allergies may be great and usually becomes worse as a dog ages.

Hair loss and skin irritation are the two most common signs that mimic a number of other conditions. Contact a veterinarian as soon as possible to determine the origin of the problem. Your veterinarian may recommend tests such as skin scrapings, blood tests and/or allergy testing in order to confirm the diagnosis and choose the correct treatment.

The following suggestions may help provide comfort for your dog until a diagnosis can be made.

141

How to Improve Comfort

A. Contact your veterinarian as early as possible. Untreated skin conditions may lead to serious complications. Medications are available to alleviate skin irritations and hasten healing. Your veterinarian can also determine if your dog's skin condition is one that could be caused by underlying disease or if it could be contagious to humans.

B. Shampooing your dog will likely provide temporary relief from its symptoms. Use a shampoo for dogs (moisturizing shampoo is best). While restraining your dog, lather the pet and let stand for 15-20 minutes. Rinse well with warm tap water. Next, mix 1 tablespoon of bath oil (e.g., Alpha Keri®) with 2 quarts of warm tap water. Then pour the bath-oil mixture over the dog's coat, being careful not to get any in its eyes. Let the coat dry naturally. Consult your veterinarian for the proper type of shampoo and for specific instructions.

C. If your dog is biting itself, you may need to apply an Elizabethan collar to prevent more damage to the skin. See pages 239-240 on how to make and use an Elizabethan collar.

STRAINING

When a dog stains to go to urinate or defecate, you can assume there is a problem. There are several conditions that cause straining that are worth mentioning, such as prostatic disease, bladder irritations or blockages, colitis, and constipation.

When the male dog's prostate gland becomes enlarged (e.g., from aging changes, the development of cysts, infection or cancer), the result is often a variety of complications. An enlarged prostate gland can compress the rectum, resulting in straining during bowel movements. The enlargement can become so severe that constipation can develop. It may also put pressure on the urethra, causing difficulty urinating.

Bladder irritations or blockages can cause a dog to strain and/or urinate without control. Usually the intervals between urinations become shorter and may result in accidents in the house. Other symptoms include blood in the urine and urgency. Causes of irritations include bladder infections, bladder crystals and/or stones. Bladder stones, tumors, and prostatic enlargement may partially obstruct the outflow of urine, causing the leakage of urine around the problem as pressure in the bladder increases. These changes can be observed in dogs of any age but become more common as dogs get older. If your dog is not producing urine, contact your veterinarian immediately.

Colitis is inflammation of the colon. An affected dog may strain after or during a bowel movement, and the straining can often be mistaken for constipation. A dog experiencing colitis may have blood or mucous in its stool. The stools may be soft in consistency and larger in volume. If no bowel movement is produced, check under your dog's tail for evidence of soft stool pasted to the hair. Your dog may need to go outside often and may show urgency in its need.

Colitis has many different causes, including allergic reactions, dietary indiscretions, foreign bodies, parasitic infestations and cancers. Although not all causes of colitis are serious, the amount of discomfort the dog feels can be great. Aging dogs may be more sensitive to dietary changes, which can lead to colitis. Colitis which recurs or is chronic may be a sign that there is a serious problem, and the problem should be investigated.

143

Straining is usually the hallmark sign of constipation. Constipation in dogs refers to their inability to defecate over a period of a few days. The causes of constipation are many. Diet irregularities such as the ingestion of hair, grass, bone, fabric, or wood can cause impactions. Lack of fiber will contribute to constipation. Certain drugs can slow the bowels or cause hardened stools. Any condition that causes pain while pushing to defecate can cause the dog to go too long between bowel movements. Examples of these conditions include anal sac abscesses, pelvic fractures, back pain, and tumors in the colon. Hernias around the rectum and enlarged prostate glands may also cause the stool to accumulate. Any illness that causes dehydration may predispose the dog to constipation. Metabolic diseases, such as hypothyroidism may also have an effect on the bowels. Spinal cord injuries and degeneration impair the sensations of having bowel movements, and may prevent a dog from pushing during a bowel movement.

If the constipation starts to interfere with the electrolyte balance and causes inflammation inside the colon, other signs of illness may be seen, such as vomiting and depression. Often the dog will develop diarrhea while constipated; the diarrhea can pass around the obstruction of hard stool, which means that the dog can still be constipated even if diarrhea is present. Do not mistake small amounts of diarrhea for a successful bowel movement.

Constipation by itself can have serious consequences if not corrected promptly. The stool inside becomes harder and drier with time, which makes removal more difficult. The retention of stool can result in a lack of appetite, vomiting, and dehydration. Prolonged retention of stool can also cause permanent enlargement of the colon and nerve damage to the colon.

If a bowel movement has not been produced within 48 hours, consult a veterinarian. Usually constipation can be diagnosed with an examination, though the cause of the constipation may require additional testing. Blood tests can be performed to rule out disease processes that could result in colitis. X-rays or a colonoscopy may be necessary to examine the bowels further. (A colonoscopy is a diagnostic test that uses a fiberoptic scope to look directly at the inside of the colon. It can also be used to retrieve an object or perform a biopsy.) Once the cause of the constipation has been determined, treatment is directed at curing that problem.

Constipation can be treated most effectively by a veterinarian. A series of delicate enemas and sedation may be required to relieve an impaction. Correction of dehydration is also important to prevent further complications, especially in an aging pet.

Dietary changes, such as increasing fiber, can help reduce the chance of a recurrence, regardless of the cause. A dog with constipation should be walked more often and longer to provide more of an opportunity to have a bowel movement.

How to Improve Comfort

A. Observe your dog for urine output or diarrhea. Your dog should be able to excrete at least small amounts of urine and should have normal bowel movements.

B. If no urine production is detected, the situation is urgent; your dog's urinary system may be blocked, and blockage is life threatening.

1. Contact a veterinarian immediately.

2. Monitor your dog's vital signs until a veterinarian can be reached.

3. Keep your dog warm by placing a 2-liter soda bottle filled with warm water (not hot water) against your dog.

4. To prevent additional discomfort and possible rupture of the bladder, avoid lifting the dog around its abdomen.

C. Even if urine is being produced, consult a veterinarian as soon as possible for diagnosis and treatment of other causes of straining. See pages 77-78 (Colitis) and pages 79-80 (Constipation).

VOMITING

It is not normal for a dog to vomit. If vomiting does not stop, or if there are other signs of illness associated with it, the condition should be of concern. There are many causes of vomiting in the dogs, including dietary indiscretions, infections, exposure to toxins, an obstruction, and parasites. Older dogs are at higher risk of other causes of vomiting such as intolerance to certain drugs, digestive ulceration, diabetes, kidney disease, liver disease, electrolyte imbalances, inflammation, cancers, constipation, pancreatitis, inner ear disorders, infections, and other metabolic problems. Aging muscles and nerves of the throat and esophagus (the tube from the mouth to the stomach) may promote regurgitation or gagging (i.e., dry heaves).

Observing the particular circumstances surrounding the vomiting will aid in determining the cause. Be able to tell your veterinarian whether your dog is on any medications (and know which ones). Describe the frequency of the vomiting and how long after a meal it occurred. You should note whether the vomited matter contains undigested food or whether it is clear or yellow. Also note if there is any blood in it. (The blood may have a coffee-ground appearance due to the mixing of blood with digestive juices.) Note whether the vomited matter has any unusual smell, and note the severity of the vomiting. (E.g., is it projectile vomiting?) Also note any other signs of illness, and describe them to the dog's veterinarian.

Diagnosis of the cause of vomiting is made through an examination by a veterinarian. Testing may be required to further investigate the cause. Blood tests, X-rays, ultrasound, endoscopy, and sometimes even exploratory surgery, may be necessary to obtain a proper diagnosis.

One of the goals in helping a dog that is vomiting is to comfort the pet and lessen the symptoms until the dog can be examined by a veterinarian. First, make sure you withhold food and water when your dog has been vomiting. If your dog continues to eat and drink, in all likelihood the vomiting will continue. The appropriate length of time to withhold food and water will depend upon the health of your dog and the seriousness of the illness. Two to four hours is probably appropriate for a normal, healthy dog, whereas an hour or two is the maximum time for an older or sick dog. (Ask your veterinarian before withholding food and water from a dog that is unhealthy or has any medical condition.) This brief time without food and water gives the digestive tract a chance to rest.

How to Assist and Improve Comfort

A. To assist the veterinarian, note the frequency and substance of the vomiting. Is the food undigested or is the vomitus watery? Note how long after a meal the vomiting occurred.

B. If your dog is vomiting, withhold food and water for 2-4 hours. (But if your dog has diabetes or any other type of illness or medical condition, consult your veterinarian first before withholding food and water.) Do not withhold food and water from a puppy or elderly dog for more than 2 hours. If symptoms persist, worsen or return within this 2-4 hour period, contact your veterinarian.

C. When you do resume feeding your dog, prepare a 50/50 mixture of boiled hamburger (drain off the water and fat) and plain cooked rice. Appropriate feedings are as follows:
    (1) 1/4 cup of the mixture 4 times per day for small dogs,
    (2) 1/2 cup of the mixture 4 times per day for medium dogs,
    (3) 3/4 cup of the mixture 4 times per day for large dogs.
    Your veterinarian may wish to adjust the servings or may recommend a prescription diet.

D. Resume normal feeding as directed by your veterinarian.

WEAKNESS AND COLLAPSE

Weakness and collapse are symptoms that may denote a problem of great significance. Weakness and collapse may be caused by a number of disorders, including heart disease, seizures, lung disease, internal bleeding, trauma, infections, poisonings, urinary blockages, bloat/gastric torsion (twisted stomach), anemia, shock, organ failure, or almost any other disease process. However, there are several problems aging dogs experience in which weakness or collapse may be the first sign. These include internal bleeding, bloat, Addison's disease (hypoadrenocorticism) and shock.

The causes of internal bleeding are many. In young dogs, trauma is the main cause, but in aging dogs, the blood loss may be due to hemorrhage from tumors or ulcers, destruction of red blood cells and lack of platelets to clot blood (e.g., from an autoimmune disease). You should suspect internal bleeding if your dog's strength deteriorates and its gums turn pale, and you should contact your veterinarian immediately.

When a dog's stomach becomes distended by gas (a condition called "bloat") or when the stomach actually twists and cuts off the blood supply to the stomach (called "twisted stomach", "gastric volvulus" or "gastric torsion"), the result is extreme pain. Bloat and twisted stomach are conditions of unknown origin. Deep-chested dogs (e.g., Great Danes, Saint Bernards, Weimaraners) are more predisposed than others to these conditions. Some veterinarians recommend that deep-chested dogs not be exercised shortly after they have eaten as a precautionary measure for avoiding bloat and twisted stomach. The symptoms of bloat include inability to belch, unsuccessful attempts to vomit, severe pain, restlessness, weakness, collapse, and/or distended stomach. If an affected dog does not receive immediate veterinary care, the condition is usually fatal.

Addison's disease is a condition whereby the dog's adrenal glands produce too little cortisol. The condition can be corrected with proper medication, but without medication it can be fatal. Early symptoms include weakness and collapse, and a host of generalized health conditions, such as vomiting, trembling, shaking, etc.

Shock is an event that accompanies some diseases and injuries. It occurs when a series of compensatory mechanisms in the body goes

148

awry. Problems that can cause shock include overwhelming infections, trauma, severe vomiting and diarrhea, blood loss, and any other serious medical situation. During the shock process, the body cannot keep up with the mixed signals that are being relayed. The body has a relative loss of blood due to changes in circulation or from bleeding. Changes in blood pressure shunt blood from vital organs such as the heart, lungs, liver, kidneys and brain to other less important areas of the body. Early signs include weakness or even collapse. Other changes include decreased vital signs: body temperature may fall; breathing may be shallow; and pulse may be weak. The dog's feet, tail, and ears may feel cold to the touch. The result can be fatal if not treated early.

Weakness that persists or gets worse should be considered a medical emergency. Any time your dog collapses, seek treatment immediately. The following suggestions will help keep your dog comfortable until the pet can be seen by a veterinarian.

How To Improve Comfort

A. Contact a veterinarian immediately. Weakness and collapse may be signs of a life-threatening condition.

B. Keep your dog warm by placing a 2-liter soda bottle filled with warm water (not hot water) against your dog. See illustration on page 135. Cover your dog with a towel or blanket.

C. Monitor your dog's vital signs (temperature, pulse and respirations) every 15 minutes and record the information. Try to keep your dog's temperature within the range of 101-103 degrees Fahrenheit. If your dog's temperature rises above 103 degrees Fahrenheit, remove the warm soda bottle. If your dog's temperature falls below 100 degrees, place an additional warm-water soda bottle against the pet, but make sure the water is not hot, and make sure the bottle is against your dog and not on top of or underneath your dog.

D. **If your dog is unconscious**, check for breathing by watching your dog's chest rise and fall.

E. **If your dog is breathing**, proceed to Step G. Do not use CPR.

F. **If your dog is not breathing,**

(1) Establish an airway by removing any debris from your dog's mouth or by moving the tongue from the back of the throat. Check for breathing by watching your dog's chest rise and fall. If your dog is breathing, proceed to Step G, and do not use CPR.

(2) If your dog is not breathing, lay your dog on its side (and throughout these procedures keep your dog on its side). Check for a pulse by placing a hand over your dog's chest just behind the shoulder blade to feel the heartbeat or by placing a hand in the groin area to feel the femoral pulse.

(3) Cup your hand(s) over your dog's nose and mouth to form a seal, with an opening for your mouth. Deliver 1 breath into your pet every 2 seconds. If the seal is proper, you should observe your dog's chest rise and fall.

(4) If after you have delivered 5 breaths your dog does not show signs of breathing on its own or signs of consciousness, and there is no heartbeat, then have a helper place a hand just behind your dog's shoulder blades, and apply gentle but firm compressions downward (compressing 1/2 to 1 inch for a small dog up to as much as 2 inches for a large dog) at a rate of 2 compressions every 1 second. If a helper is not available, alternate delivering 2 breaths then 10 compressions. **Do not do any compressions if there is a pulse, no matter how faint.**

(5) Check for a pulse and breathing every 2 minutes. If there is no pulse and breathing, continue for up to 10 minutes before giving up.

G. If your dog is conscious, proceed as follows:

(1) Keep your pet calm, and avoid unnecessary stress. Do not use excessive restraint or cause excessive movement. Plan the handling of your dog to minimize stress. Never hold your dog tightly.

(2) Lay your dog upright (i.e., belly down). (If your dog is on

its back or side, there is extra pressure on the chest, making it harder for your pet to breathe.)

H.   Seek immediate veterinary care.

WEIGHT GAIN

Weight gain is common in older dogs. Perhaps as many as one quarter to one half of all dogs are overweight. Both large and small dogs are at risk for obesity. In general, as a dog ages, its caloric intake needs to be decreased slightly because of reduced activity. The causes of weight gain may be as simple as decreased activity and an increased consumption of food, or consumption of food high in fat and calories. Also, drugs such as cortisone and phenobarbitol may make dogs feel more hungry. Boredom may also encourage overeating. An older dog also has a decreased metabolic rate, which can contribute to weight gain. Finally, disease processes can either directly or indirectly have an effect on a dog's weight. For example, degenerative joint disease can lead to an increased weight gain by decreasing an animal's ability to exercise. Another disease, hypothyroidism, is a hormonal condition which slows metabolism so that even if the dog is not eating much, it is unable to lose weight and may continue to gain weight. Cushing's disease may also cause the dog to gain weight.

Some weight gain may appear to be more sudden due to the enlargement of an organ or the accumulation of fluid in places it normally is not seen, such as in the abdomen (ascites). This type of weight gain is of urgent concern.

Any sudden or substantial weight gain signifies a medical problem. If you cannot feel the rib cage, cannot define the dog's waist, or if there is rounding of the belly, or if there are fat deposits over the hips, your dog may be overweight and you should contact a veterinarian for a consultation.

Abnormal weight gain should be of serious concern because of the role it plays in a variety of medical problems. Abnormal weight gain tends to make a medical situation worse and predisposes a dog to various diseases. A dog that is overweight has a higher incidence of arthritis or degenerative joint disease because of excess stress on the joints. The increased accumulation of fat also compromises breathing by putting undue pressure on vital structures in the chest. Increased fat acts as an insulator, interfering with temperature regulation and resulting in a greater potential for heat stroke. Obesity also affects the immune system, resulting in increased risk of infection, and affects sugar metabolism, making a dog susceptible to diabetes. And overweight dogs have a higher risk of anesthetic problems during surgeries.

Determining the cause of the weight gain and then getting help to resolve the problem will help extend your dog's lifespan and help your dog to be more comfortable.

How to Prevent Weight Gain and Improve Comfort

A. If your dog can be lifted easily, weigh the dog on a bathroom scale by weighing yourself with your dog and then subtracting your weight from the total weight. Weigh your dog regularly (i.e., weekly), and record the weight to note whether the weight is increasing over time. If so, consult your veterinarian for recommendations. If weighing your dog is impractical, ask your veterinarian about visiting the veterinarian's office for use of a walk-on pet scale.

B. If your dog is overweight, contact a veterinarian for a balanced reducing dog food that is low in calories and high in fiber. You should avoid bulk generic foods which may not provide balanced nutrition.

C. Keep a record of the brand of food and amount of food your dog consumes. Also keep track of the frequency of feedings.

D. Feed your dog several small meals daily (3-4 times daily).

E. If you have more than one dog, feed the overweight dog by itself to decrease overeating due to competition.

F. Keep your dog out of the kitchen and the dining room.

G. Some veterinarians suggest adding canned green beans or carrots to a dog's diet to add healthful bulk and help make a dog feel full.

H. Decrease the portions you feed your dog if you give your dog any treats.

I. If you do feed your dog treats, choose ones that are low in calories and fat. Feed the treats in smaller portions, and include the amount of calories from treats in your dog's daily allowance. Treats should be less than 10% of the calories of your dog's diet.

Note that a large dog biscuit may contain more than 100 calories. Consult your veterinarian regarding appropriate treats for your dog.

J. Study your dog's habits closely for amount of food consumed, vomiting, diarrhea, water consumption, weakness, depression, and any other unusual changes. Report these changes to your veterinarian to help pinpoint a medical cause.

K. Develop an appropriate exercise program for your dog with the guidance of your veterinarian. (See page 45-48.)

    1. Increase your dog's activity gradually to lessen the potential for injuries.

    2 Exercise does not need to be rigorous in order to be beneficial. In general, two walks daily for 15 minutes will help burn calories.

    3. Select exercises that are appropriate for your dog's condition. For example, if your dog suffers from joint problems, consider swimming as an alternative to running.

    4. Record the type of exercise and the frequency of exercise.

L. Consult with a veterinarian before making any changes in your dog's nutrition or exercise.

WEIGHT LOSS

Weight loss can occur in dogs of any age but is of particular concern in an older dog. Weight loss is considered significant when the total decrease in weight is greater than 10% of the dog's average weight. Signs of weight loss or being underweight include the visibility of the rib cage, spine and pelvic bones. There may also be a loss of muscle mass, and the dog's waist may be very thin.

There are many causes of weight loss, including decreased food intake, metabolic problems, illness, parasites or even environmental conditions. Decreased food intake can result from a variety of causes, including dental pain or decreased appetite from illness. Inadequate intake of food can also occur if a dog is underfed, is fed poor quality food, is fed spoiled food, or is exercised excessively. Digestive problems, such as vomiting and diarrhea, do not allow a dog to utilize the food that is available and therefore have the same effect as decreased food intake. Other illnesses, such as chronic diseases, cancers, fever, and heart failure may also increase a dog's metabolism or cause loss of nutrients and a decrease in weight. Parasitic infestations can rob your dog of nutrition and cause substantial weight loss. Environmental stresses, such as excessive cold, also can cause weight loss.

When a dog losses substantial body weight and the bones of the ribs, spine, shoulders, and hips begin to show, the condition is called emaciation, and it is serious. Further weight loss with weakness and confusion is called cachexia and may be a terminal condition.

How to Prevent Weight Loss and Improve Comfort

A. If your dog can be lifted easily, weigh the dog on a bathroom scale by weighing yourself with your dog and then subtracting your weight from the total weight. Weigh your dog regularly (i.e., weekly), and record the weight to note whether the weight is decreasing over time. If the accumulated weight loss is more than 10% of the dog's normal weight, consult your dog's veterinarian for recommendations. If weighing your dog is impractical, ask your veterinarian about visiting the veterinarian's office for use of a walk-on pet scale. Report any decrease in weight to your veterinarian.

B. Provide your dog with a balanced dog food. You should avoid bulk generic foods that may not provide balanced nutrition. Consult your veterinarian.

C. Upon recommendation from your veterinarian, provide your dog with a multi-vitamin.

D. Collect a stool specimen for your veterinarian to check for parasites.

E. Study your dog's habits closely to determine the amount of food and water consumed and to note any regurgitation, vomiting, diarrhea, weakness, depression, or any other unusual changes.

F. Limit your dog's activity until your dog can be examined.

PART 4

CREATIVE IDEAS TO COPE WITH THE PROBLEMS OF AGING

INTRODUCTION TO CREATIVE IDEAS

Dogs over five years of age can have special needs and require special care, and sometimes creative ideas are necessary to provide the best care for your dog. The creative ideas described in this chapter are designed to give you the resources to cope with adverse changes associated with aging. The first chapters include topics such as proper handling, how to help your dog get up and down, and how to provide safe transportation. The following sections deal with general care, such as feeding, dental hygiene, grooming, diapering and massage. The final topics include useful procedures, such as first-aid techniques, giving medicines, and administering subcutaneous fluids.

HANDLING AGING DOGS

Hurt, sick, or older dogs may react unpredictably when there is a problem; often instinctual behavior overrides normal disposition. Some dogs may become anxious, confused, or aggressive when they are in pain or are afraid. Health conditions that tend to occur as a dog ages, such as arthritis and loss of vision or hearing can have a significant impact on the behavior and disposition of your pet.

Handling an older dog is often a challenge because if the dog struggles, it may injure itself. If your dog is frightened, is in obvious pain or is behaving aggressively, your approach and handling techniques are important. Approach an anxious dog slowly and calmly, talking quietly to the pet. Repeat "good dog," "good girl" or "good boy." If your dog has difficulty hearing, create vibration while approaching by stepping firmly so that your dog will not be startled. Approach your dog from behind to avoid being bitten. Once your dog is in hand, the pet can be lifted or positioned for further care or examination. If your dog is resisting, take care not to be too aggressive in restraining it. Older dogs with lung problems may stop breathing if stressed or if their chest is held too tightly. Older dogs may also have weakened bones, and restraining them too forcefully could cause fractures. Because many older dogs have arthritis, firm restraint may cause considerable discomfort and should be avoided. To hold your dog in place, put one arm under the dog's stomach (below the ribs) and your other hand under the dog's neck (with your dog's neck in the corner of your elbow). See the illustration on page 160. When lifting your dog, bend your knees and lift with equal pressure on both arms.

If your dog does not allow your touch and aggressively resists your direct contact, consider using a large towel or blanket instead of your hands. Place the towel or blanket over the pet, and gently gather your dog in the towel/blanket to complete the restraint. If you suspect that your dog has a fracture or a neck or back injury, take care to avoid excessive movement. Movement can be minimized by sliding your pet onto a small board or directly into a pet carrier.

If you follow the rules for basic restraint techniques, the stress during a problem will be decreased for your pet and for you.

Special Considerations for Handling Older Dogs

A. Talk to your dog calmly and quietly, unless the dog is deaf. For deaf dogs, step firmly to create vibration.

B. Be patient and gentle because older dogs become confused and scared more easily than younger dogs.

C. Avoid holding your dog too tightly because excessive pressure on your dog's chest may interfere with its breathing.

D. Do not use excessive force during restraint, and do not pull on the legs of your older dog because its bones may be fragile.

E. Arthritis may make any restraint painful. Consult your veterinarian to determine the most appropriate method for handling your dog.

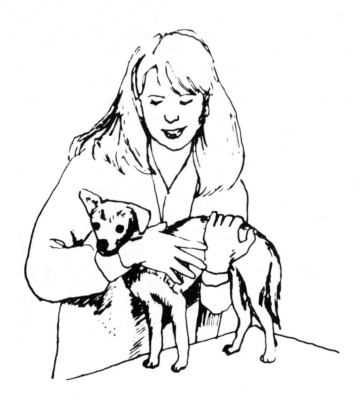

GETTING UP AND DOWN

Helping your dog to get up and down will preserve muscle strength, improve circulation, and provide ample opportunity for your dog to go to the bathroom. Frequently, older dogs experience difficulty getting up and lying down. Regardless of the cause of the difficulty, there are some techniques you can use to assist your dog. For small dogs, you can assist simply by lifting and carrying the dog as necessary. However, for medium size and large dogs, the situation is much more challenging.

Proper footing is important for dogs that have difficulty getting up and down. Slippery floors are hazardous for older dogs who cannot get the necessary traction. Provide your dog with a good surface by using nonskid throw rugs, bath mats or industrial rubber mats. Towels and blankets are soft but too slippery to be of aid.

Dogs that have difficulty rising, most commonly have problems with their hind legs. Their difficulty may be the result of arthritis pain, or it may be the result of weakness from illness or nerve degeneration. If your dog has some strength remaining in its rear quarters and has good forelimb strength, you can place a towel under the dog's abdomen to help it get up. See the illustration below:

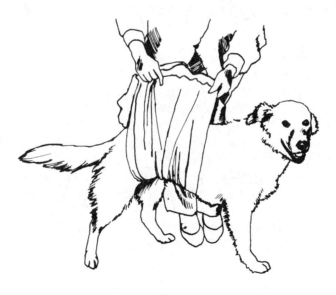

Once the towel is in place, use it as a sling, and lift by holding both ends with equal pressure. If your dog has weak legs front and back, you can help the dog get up by placing one towel between the front legs and another under your dog's abdomen. Lift the front towel first using equal pressure on both ends of the towel. Once the front end is almost up, start to lift the back towel. A cloth log carrier with a handle can be used as a substitute for a towel. Whether you use a towel or a log carrier, remember that your dog is dependent upon you for its balance, and you must be careful not to let your pet stumble and hit its nose on the ground.

Dogs that are paralyzed in their hind limbs but have good forelimb strength may benefit from special carts designed to support the hind end. These carts enable a paralyzed dog to function and enjoy activity much the same as a normal, healthy dog. They are custom made for your dog's dimensions. Note, however, that a dog with a cart should be watched closely to avoid any dangerous situations (e.g., stairs or hazardous terrain).

Dogs with forelimb difficulties can be helped up by running a towel between the front legs, then lifting with equal pressure. (This method may be facilitated by grasping and gently pulling up on the collar at the same time.) See the illustrations on page 163.

While small dogs may be easy to lift and carry, larger dogs may be more difficult. To lift and move a medium size to large dog that does not have the strength to help itself, put one arm under your dog's stomach (below the ribs) and the other hand under your dog's neck (with your dog's neck in the corner of your elbow). When lifting your dog, bend your knees and lift with equal pressure on both arms. If your strength does not permit you to lift your dog, tuck a blanket under your dog or roll your dog onto a blanket and pull the dog on the blanket or have someone lift opposite corners.

In addition to difficulty rising, some dogs have difficulty lying down. When this occurs, it is usually because there is an arthritic condition that causes pain during the process. These dogs benefit from helping them tuck their back legs underneath them. They may also benefit from having something to brace against when trying to lie down, such as the support of your legs. Placing large soft pillows around the dog may allow for a graduated transition from the up to the down position.

Contact your veterinarian if there is any change in your dog's ability to get up and down. Also contact a veterinarian if you are unable to move your dog.

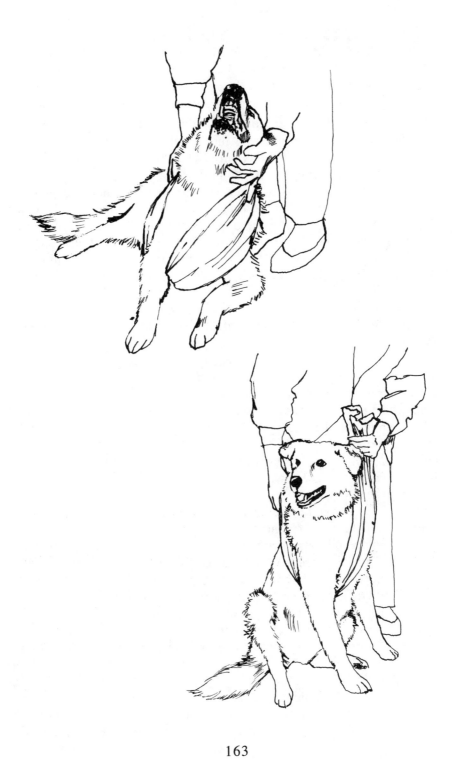

TRANSPORTATION

Transporting older dogs is sometimes problematic. Older dogs may have difficulty getting into a vehicle because of arthritis, weakness, pain or decreased flexibility. They may become anxious or confused about entering and traveling in a car.

For your own safety, when you are driving, your dog should never be in your lap or on the floor near the car's pedals. If there is no passenger-side airbag, your dog can ride in the front passenger seat; otherwise, your dog should ride in the back. Restrain and secure your pet with a leash or a special dog safety belt, or, for a small dog, you may place it in a carrier or have a helper hold the pet. For your dog's safety, never allow the pet to ride with its head outside the window or with its paws on the window's edge. Never allow a small dog to ride on the back window ledge, and never drive with your dog in the open bed of a truck.

A small dog should be transported in a pet carrier to provide safety and comfort. Obtain a pet carrier that has a removable top. If a pet carrier is not available, use a corrugated cardboard box of an appropriate size. A carrier or box that opens at the top rather than the side is preferable because a dog can be put in and taken out without pushing or pulling. Slide your hands under your dog to lift. Take care to support your dog's entire body as you lift and place your dog into the carrier. Place towels around your dog to keep the pet from sliding in the pet carrier.

If your dog can be easily lifted, it should be placed in the back seat of the car. If your dog is not too large for you to carry by yourself, place one arm under its stomach (below the ribs) and the other hand under its neck (with your dog's neck in the corner formed by your elbow). See the illustration on page 160. When lifting your dog, bend your knees and lift with equal pressure on both arms. Towels or blankets should be packed on the floor to prevent your dog from falling off of the seat and being injured.

There are special guidelines to follow if your dog has been injured. In the event of an emergency, even a friendly dog may bite when it is in pain. Therefore, apply a muzzle if your dog is not having difficulty breathing and has not been vomiting. However, do not use a muzzle if your dog has a flat face (e.g., a pug, boxer, English bulldog, etc.). For spinal cord and bone injuries, the risk of

164

additional injury from moving an injured dog is substantial. The ideal carrying method is to slide the dog onto a plywood board and then secure the pet with a blanket. If a board is not available, use a blanket instead. You will need someone to assist you in carrying the board or blanket. If you do use a board, make sure that it will fit in the vehicle you plan to use for transport. A small dog with a spine or bone injury can be placed in a pet carrier as described above.

For emergencies other than spinal cord and bone injuries, you may still need to use a board or large blanket (as detailed immediately above) if your dog is too large for you to carry by yourself. If your dog is not too large for you to carry by yourself, place one arm under your dog's stomach (below the ribs) and your other hand under its neck (with your dog's neck in the corner formed by your elbow). See the illustration on page 160. When lifting your dog, bend your knees and lift with equal pressure on both arms.

If you suspect that your dog is going into shock, proceed as follows: (1) If your dog is in pain, you may wish to use a muzzle. However, use a muzzle only if your dog is not having difficulty breathing and has not been vomiting. If at any time your dog has difficulty breathing, remove the muzzle. Also, do not use a muzzle if your dog has a flat face (e.g., a pug, boxer, English bulldog, etc.). (2) Lay your dog on the seat of the car. (3) Pack blankets around your dog to keep your pet warm. If you are concerned that your dog may slide off of the seat onto the floor, pack the floor area with a pillow or blankets. (4) Place one or two 2-liter soda bottles filled with warm water (not hot water) against your dog.

The outline below is a summary of the most important safety precautions for transporting your older dog.

Special Considerations for Transporting the Older Dog

I. For your own driving safety:

    A. Your dog should ride in the seat next to the driver (if there is no passenger side air bag) or in the back seat, but never in the driver's lap or near the pedals.

    B. Restrain and secure your pet with a leash or a special dog safety belt. For a small dog, you may wish to use a pet carrier instead, or have a helper hold the pet.

165

II. For your dog's safety:
   A. Help your dog into the car. You may need to lift or boost your aging dog making sure that your dog does not fall.
   B. Never allow your pet to ride with its head outside the window or with its paws on the window's edge.
   C. Never allow a small dog to ride on the back window ledge.
   D. Never drive with your dog in the open bed of a truck.
   E. Help your dog out of the car so it does not stumble while leaping down.
III. Transporting a dog that has injuries or is in shock:
   A. If your dog is in pain, you may wish to use a muzzle. However, use a muzzle only if your dog is not having difficulty breathing and has not been vomiting. If at any time your dog has difficulty breathing, remove the muzzle. Also, do not use a muzzle if your dog has a flat face (e.g., a pug, boxer, English bulldog, etc.).
   B. Lay your dog on the seat of the car. Pack blankets around your dog to keep the pet warm. If you are concerned that your dog may slide off of the seat onto the floor, pack the floor area with a pillow or blankets.
   C. Place one or two 2-liter soda bottles filled with warm water (not hot water) against your dog.

FEEDING

The nutritional needs of an aging dog are different from those of a younger more active dog. In general, an older dog does not require as many calories as a younger dog. The amount of protein in the diet can also be decreased. Modifications in food type, food preparation, and meal times may benefit an aging dog. Ask your veterinarian. Increased fiber in the diet may aid in digestion and prevent digestive upsets. Also, many pet food companies have good formulated diets for older dogs.

As a dog ages, the need for certain nutrients may be dictated by disease processes. For example, dogs with heart disease may benefit from a prescription diet low in sodium to decrease blood pressure. Dogs with severe kidney disease may benefit from foods restricted in protein to decrease the work load of the kidneys. Your veterinarian can best advise which diet is optimal for your dog based on its health. Also, older dogs in general have an increased need for vitamins A, E, and B, and you should ask your veterinarian about an appropriate vitamin supplement. An older dog's hair coat will also benefit from zinc and fatty acids provided in some supplements. Dogs should never be fed people food or people vitamins unless under the instruction of a veterinarian.

There are some feeding preparation techniques that may benefit your dog's health. Dogs with decreased appetites may be encouraged to eat by warming their food to increase the smell and palatability. Addition of water, bouillon, clam juice or garlic may make dry food more tempting. Any changes in food preparation should be gradually introduced to avoid digestive upsets. Ask your veterinarian about trying different appropriate diets to encourage your dog's appetite.

Make sure that your dog's food is fresh. Replace old food as needed rather than waiting until your dog has eaten all of the old food. And make sure that your dog's water is fresh. Fresh water should never be withheld from an older dog unless it is vomiting. Refusal to eat or drink may signify a serious medical problem and is cause for contacting a veterinarian.

Some dogs are more likely to eat better in the presence of other animals because of the threat of competition. Others can benefit from having you stay and talk to them during feeding time, and others may benefit from hand feeding.

Most dogs with medical conditions benefit from the feeding of several small feedings per day. This helps the digestion of foods and provides a continual source of energy throughout the day. Several smaller meals may also help dogs on reducing diets feel more satisfied.

Some dogs with medical problems will have an increased appetite. It is important in this case to report the increase to your veterinarian and be careful of weight gain.

As mentioned earlier, a decreased appetite may be a sign of a medical problem. Consult your veterinarian for a diagnosis and advice. In addition to treating any underlying condition or disease, a veterinarian can, if necessary, prescribe medicines and vitamins to stimulate your dog's appetite.

As mentioned above, dogs should never be fed people food or people vitamins unless under the instruction of a veterinarian. Certain people foods are difficult for a dog to digest and can result in conditions such as pancreatitis (inflammation of the pancreas), colitis (inflammation of the colon), and gastroenteritis (inflammation of the stomach and intestines). Some of these diseases can be life threatening. Do not supplement a dog's diet without a veterinarian's advice because wrong supplementation can cause urinary tract problems, metabolic problems, and even mineralization of the kidneys. Never oversupplement your dog's diet with vitamin D or fish liver oil. Excess can cause bone disease as well as digestive upset.

Never feed dogs cat food. Cat food lacks the balance of nutrients essential for healthy dogs. Also, it may cause diarrhea, or the high fat content may promote obesity. Also, never feed dogs milk. Milk can cause digestive problems such as diarrhea.

Never feed a dog raw fish. Raw fish causes a thiamine deficiency which may result in loss of appetite, a hunched and painful stance, and possibly convulsions. Even if it is cooked, never feed a dog a diet of fish exclusively. Never feed a dog foods that contain rancid fats or excess polyunsaturated fats because they can cause a vitamin E deficiency, leading to a variety of muscle diseases. Never feed your dog bones or chocolates.

Below is a summary of the major points discussed in the paragraphs above.

Special Considerations in Feeding Older Dogs

A. Report any decrease or increase in your dog's appetite to your veterinarian.

B. With the advice of a veterinarian, choose the correct food type according to your dog's age, weight, and medical status.

C. Fresh water should always be available. Never withhold water from an older dog unless it is vomiting.

D. Make sure food is fresh.

E. Never feed your dog people food unless approved by a veterinarian.

F. Make diet changes gradually.

G. Consider warming food to increase palatability.

H. Consider adding water, bouillon, clam juice, or garlic to enhance taste.

I. A different diet may increase interest in food.

J. Serving food in the presence of other animals may increase appetite because of competition.

K. Human companionship through petting and talking or hand feeding may encourage your dog to eat.

L. Feed several small meals per day.

M. Never feed your dog cat food. Cat food lacks the balance of nutrients essential for healthy dogs. Also, it may cause diarrhea, or the high fat content may promote obesity.

N. Never feed your dog milk. Milk can cause digestive problems such as diarrhea.

O. Do not supplement diets without a veterinarian's advice. Wrong supplementation can cause urinary tract problems, metabolic problems and even mineralization of the kidneys.

P. Never feed your dog raw fish. Raw fish causes a thiamine deficiency which may result in loss of appetite, a hunched and painful stance, and possibly convulsions. Even if it is cooked, never feed your dog a diet of fish exclusively.

Q. Never feed your dog foods that contain rancid fats or excess polyunsaturated fats because they can cause a vitamin E deficiency leading to a variety of muscle diseases.

R.   Never oversupplement your dog's diet with vitamin D or fish liver oil. Excess can cause bone disease as well as digestive upset.

S.   Never feed your dog bones or chocolates.

GROOMING

Grooming is important in maintaining good physical and mental health for the dog. For a variety of reasons, older dogs may require more grooming. Debilitation associated with illnesses and aging can cause an older dog to become soiled or matted more often. And older dogs are more affected by minor grooming problems that most younger dogs can more easily tolerate (e.g., toenail problems or hair interfering with sight or hearing).

A dog should be kept combed and brushed daily in order to remove dirt and shedding hair from the coat. This daily attention also will increase circulation and make you aware of any lumps or bumps developing on the skin. In breeds with long hair, care for an aging dog is easier if its coat is kept short. If clipping your dog's hair is not possible or desirable, at least be sure to keep the hair trimmed around the eyes, ears, mouth, and feet. Keeping the hair away from the eyes, may allow a dog with failing vision to see better by allowing more light into the eyes. Hair should be removed from around, but not inside, the ear canal to promote better hearing and prevent infection. Do not pull hair from inside your dog's ear canal because that can make your dog prone to infection. Hair should be trimmed from the mouth to help keep this area clean. Hair growing between the toes, or hair growing between the pads should be trimmed to prevent matting. Hair should also be trimmed away from the rectum and genitals to provide better hygiene and to facilitate ease of cleaning those areas.

A dog should not be bathed more often than once every two weeks unless recommended by a veterinarian. In general, increased bathing may remove the oils from the coat and lessen the skin's defenses to infection. An older dog should be bathed with a shampoo to match its skin type. Human shampoos are not usually suited for a dog's skin (because they have a different pH balance). Consult your veterinarian for the shampoo that best suits your dog.

The process of bathing may become more difficult as your dog gets older. Lifting your dog may cause your pet pain, especially if your dog has arthritis. Standing for a bath may also be difficult. A walk-in shower with a spray nozzle is the most convenient method of bathing larger breed dogs. A bath towel or mat may be placed in the bottom of the shower or tub to provide traction for your dog to prevent slipping. During warmer weather, a dog can be bathed outside using a hose hook-up to a sink where warm water can be obtained. The hose can be stretched outside through a door for the bath. Never bathe a dog in cold water; it can cause hypothermia and muscle soreness. If a whole body bath is not required, only wash the soiled area. It is important to keep urine and stool off the coat to prevent infection and sores from developing. Any time you see urine or stool on the hair coat, wash the area immediately with warm water. Be sure to rinse your dog well. After bathing your dog, be sure to dry your dog properly to prevent chilling and to ensure that the undercoat dries. Drying can be done using a hair dryer on a low setting or by vigorous towel rubbing.

Your dog's eyes, ears, and mouth require special attention. Any wetness around the eyes, ears or mouth should be dried immediately in order to prevent an infection from developing. A special ear hygiene solution can be prescribed by your veterinarian to provide twice weekly ear care to help prevent infections. Dental care may require more time as your dog ages. Your veterinarian may recommend teeth brushing or special solutions to apply to the teeth or gums to prevent or treat disorders. See pages 192-194.

Toenails should be trimmed as often as necessary. An aging dog may not wear down the nails as well as a younger more active dog. Long nails cause a dog to stand improperly, creating unnatural stress on bones and ligaments, thereby causing pain or aggravating arthritis. Nails left long can also become ingrown and infected, sometimes requiring surgery to correct.

By keeping your dog well groomed you will help prevent problems from developing. The grooming process will also help keep you up-to-date with changes in your dog and will help keep your dog comfortable. The outline below provides a summary of grooming procedures discussed above.

I. Materials Needed

A. Pet shampoo

B. Toenail trimmers

C. Scissors or clippers

D. Ear hygiene solution

E. Dental care products (toothbrush, toothpaste, hygiene spray)

II. Guidelines for Grooming Older Dogs

A. Comb or brush your dog daily.

B. Check for lumps and bumps while brushing.

C. Wipe any discharge away from around your dog's eyes.

D. Clean your dog's ears twice weekly using an ear hygiene solution approved by your veterinarian.

E. Practice dental hygiene using a toothpaste or hygiene solution recommended by your veterinarian.

F. Keep your dog's toenails trimmed.

G. Trim hair from around your dog's eyes.

H. Trim hair from around the tail area and genitals.

I. Bathe your dog with warm water as needed, but not more often than once every two weeks.

J. Use partial baths to wash small soiled areas.

K. Never bath your dog in cold water. Make sure you rinse off all of the soap, and then dry your dog well with a towel or hair dryer on low setting.

BEDDING

Providing appropriate bedding for dogs as they age will increase their comfort. An aging dog experiencing arthritis, incontinence, or chronic diseases will benefit tremendously from proper bedding. Also, an older dog may also have difficultly regulating its body temperature, and bedding may be helpful in that regard because it serves to insulate your dog's body from cold floors.

The most important feature of a good bed is cleanliness. Make sure that the bedding you select is easy to wash. Examples of appropriate bedding include folded comforters, commercial stuffed beds with removable, waterproof covers, and rubber mats covered with a blanket or towels. Foam and similar material should be avoided unless a waterproof covering is available. Waterbeds are acceptable if they are carefully monitored for proper temperature. The bed should be large enough to allow your dog to stretch out and lie flat. Its thickness depends on the type of material used, but it should provide soft padding and insulation from the floor. Soft padding is important to prevent bed sores from developing.

A variety of aids can be used if your dog is incontinent and leaks urine while in bed. A diaper or special pants may be applied to your dog as described on pages 177-178, or an absorbable pad may be placed under your dog to remove moisture away from its skin. Diapers and absorbent pads must be replaced promptly whenever they get wet because they can quickly become extreme irritants. Washing the bedding may be facilitated by having spare bedding available, especially if frequent soiling occurs. Bedding may also be protected by placing plastic (e.g., a plastic trash bag) on top of the bedding and then placing a towel on top of the plastic. (Note, however that plastic can make the bed slip and slide, and keeping the plastic in place may be difficult. A waterproof bed liner may work better than the plastic.) When bedding gets soiled, it should be washed immediately. Urine and stool saturated bedding promotes infection and bed sores.

Your dog's bed should be situated in a draft-free, dry, well-ventilated area. This area should be in a well-supervised area of the house to facilitate interaction and observation of your dog's habits. Try to avoid dark, damp basements. Your dog's food and water should be near the bed to provide easy access.

If your dog likes to sleep in your bed but has difficulty

jumping up onto the bed, you might consider putting a stepstool beside the bed. Smaller dogs may be lifted onto or off of a bed, but by creating a means for your dog to come and go at will under its own power, your dog will have greater access to food and water, toys or anything else. If your dog is too debilitated to make use of a stepstool, you may wish to consider building a plywood ramp; but make sure the ramp is at a low angle, and make sure it has a rail on both sides that your dog can balance against.

Consult your veterinarian if your dog has a special bedding need.

Special Considerations for Bedding for Older Dogs
A. Keep all bedding clean.
B. Make sure the bedding provides adequate padding plus good insulation.
C. Provide a bed large enough for your dog to lie flat.
D. Locate the bed in a draft-free, dry, well-ventilated environment.
E. Locate bed where your dog can be closely monitored.
F. Keep food and water in close proximity.

MASSAGE

Massage is a useful therapeutic tool to aid in relaxation and improve circulation. Massage also makes you aware of any changes in your dog's skin, such as hair loss and lumps or bumps. There is no one method of massage for dogs, but most dogs tend to like circular massage patterns using the finger tips or the flat of the hand. The intensity or firmness of the massage will depend upon the dog's preference and whether the area that you are massaging is painful.

A total body massage starts at the nose and ends at the tail. Start at the nose and rub the dogs lips on both sides with a backward circular motion. Slid your hands to the ears and stroke down each ear moving from the base of the ear to the tip. Repeat this until the entire ear flap has been covered. Next stroke the forehead and continue the massage down the neck. Focus the massage on the muscles supporting the neck, and then slide your hands onto the dog's shoulders. Rub the shoulders equally on both sides. Run your hands from the shoulders down the legs stopping to gently flex and extend each joint as you pass over it all the way down to the feet. Rub between the toes, unless the dog protests. Work your way back up the legs and proceed to massage the muscles along the back. Once this is accomplished, rub over each side of the rib cage and slide your hands onto the abdomen. Gently stroke the belly working your way back to the hips. Run your hands from the hips down the legs stopping to gently flex and extend each joint as you pass over it all the way down to the feet and between the toes. Continue to the tail; a gentle backward pulling to the massage of the tail may feel good to the dog. Be careful not to lift up on the tail of an older dog that has arthritis, because the upward lift motion may cause pain.

If a dog has a problem area, you may focus the massage on that spot. For bad hips, start the massage at the lower back and slowly move down the spine all the way to the tip of the tail, and then work your way down each leg to the feet and toes. Gentle flexing and extending of each joint helps keep the joints flexible. For sore shoulders, focus on the heavy muscles of the shoulders as well as the muscles in front of and behind the shoulder blades.

Time the massage to last ten to thirty minutes. There are books and tapes available that teach other techniques of massage that may be useful. Ask your veterinarian.

176

DIAPERING

When a dog ages, there are conditions that may develop that make the dog incontinent. Depending upon the underlying cause, there may be medications to help a dog that has lost control of its bowels and/or bladder. Until medication can take effect, or if the condition is unresponsive to treatment, diapering helps decrease the stress of cleaning up messes in the house.

I. Materials Needed

A. Diapers or Depends® undergarments or sanitary feminine hygiene pads

B. Panties

C. Masking tape

D. Corn starch powder

E. Baby wipes

F. Triple antibiotic ointment

II. Technique Instructions

A. Clean your dog with baby wipes or mild soap and water.

B. Apply triple antibiotic ointment to any sore areas.

C. Lightly apply corn starch powder to the area if no breathing difficulty exists.

D. Cut a hole in the diaper for your dog's tail. Place the diaper between your dog's legs. Insert the tail through the hole.

E. Pull adhesive tabs up, and then reinforce them with masking tape. You may need to stick a small portion of tape to the hair to keep the diaper on.

F. Change the diaper as needed.

G. A pair of panties with a sanitary pad placed in the crotch may be substituted for the undergarment or diaper.

H. Commercial panties made especially for dogs can now be purchased in many pet stores.

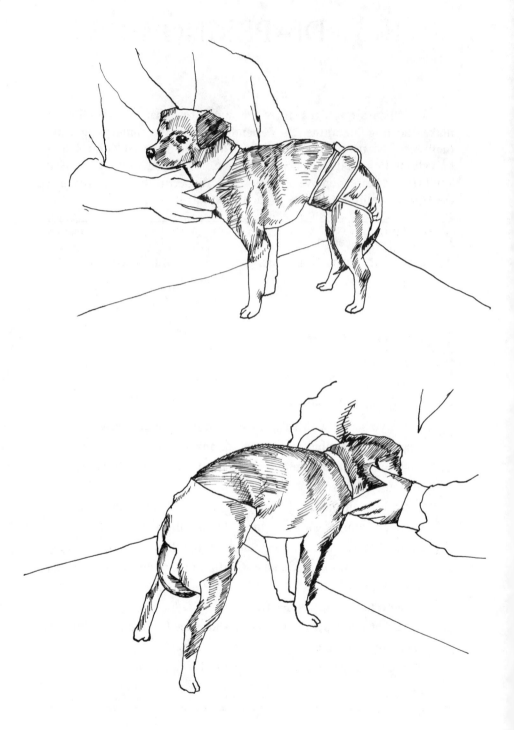

FIRST-AID TECHNIQUES

Monitoring your dog's vital signs (i.e., temperature, pulse and respirations) and performing cardiopulmonary resuscitation are two techniques that could save your dog's life. Monitoring vital signs gives you and your veterinarian a basis for evaluating your dog's progress during an illness. Changes in vital signs are an indication of changes in your dog's health status, and vital signs provide critical information for determining whether your dog's condition is getting better, staying the same or getting worse. Temperature, pulse and respirations provide significant information about shock, infection and inflammation, as well as the function of vital organs such as the heart and lungs.

Because aging dogs may suffer from a variety of problems that may cause their heart to stop temporarily, cardiopulmonary resuscitation (CPR) can be life-saving. CPR is used in the most critical situations when your dog has stopped breathing and has no pulse. When CPR is necessary, there is no time to find a veterinarian, which means that your ability to perform the technique will determine whether your dog has a chance of surviving. CPR may enable a critical dog to survive until it is transported to a veterinary hospital for additional treatment.

CPR is used to revive a dog that is not breathing and has no heartbeat. If there is a heartbeat, no matter how faint, do not perform any chest compressions. When CPR is needed, it must be performed immediately. Therefore, it is imperative that you be able to assess the need quickly and perform the technique effectively.

CPR may be used in a variety of situations in which the heart and breathing may stop, including after a seizure, choking, in heart disease, lung disease, trauma, and other crises. The following outline is a step-by-step guide for monitoring vital signs and performing CPR.

I. **Monitoring Vital Signs**
A. Taking the temperature:
    (1) Lubricate a rectal thermometer with water-soluble
        lubricating jelly or petroleum jelly. Insert the thermometer

179

gently into your dog's rectum approximately 1 inch.

    (2) Wait 2 minutes, and then remove and read the thermometer.

    (3) Normal temperature is between 101 and 103 degrees Fahrenheit.

B.   Taking the pulse:

    (1) Lay your hand just behind your dog's shoulder blade on either side of its chest and feel for the heartbeat, or

    (2) Place your hand in the groin area of your dog's abdomen and feel for the femoral pulse.

    (3) Count the beats per minute (e.g., count for 15 seconds and multiply by 4).

    (4) Normal pulse at rest should range from approximately 100 to 130 beats per minute. If your dog has been recently active or is excited, its pulse may be significantly higher.

C.   Taking respirations:

    (1) If your dog is lying quietly, watch its chest rise and fall.

    (2) Count the number of breaths your dog takes in a minute.

    (3) Normal resting respiratory rate is approximately 20 to 24 breaths per minute.

II.   Cardiopulmonary Resuscitation (CPR)

A.   Lay your dog on its side (and throughout these procedures keep your dog on its side).

B.   Check for breathing by watching your dog's chest rise and fall.

C.   **If the dog is breathing**, proceed no further. Do not use CPR.

D.   **If the dog is not breathing,**

    (1) Establish an airway by removing any debris from your dog's mouth or by moving its tongue from the back of its throat. Check for breathing by watching your dog's chest rise and fall. If your dog is breathing, proceed no further, and do not use CPR.

    (2) Check for a pulse by placing a hand over your dog's chest just behind the shoulder blade to feel the heartbeat or by placing a hand in the groin area to feel the femoral pulse.

E. **If the dog still is not breathing,**

(1) Cup your hand(s) over your dog's nose and mouth to form a seal with an opening for your mouth. Deliver 1 breath every 2 seconds. If the seal is proper, you should observe your dog's chest rise and fall.

(2) If after you have delivered 5 breaths your dog does not show signs of breathing on its own or signs of consciousness, and there is no heartbeat, then have a helper place a hand just behind your dog's shoulder blades, and apply gentle but firm compressions downward (compressing 1/2 to 1 inch for a small dog and up to as much as 2 inches for a large dog) at a rate of 2 compressions every 1 second. If a helper is not available, alternate delivering 2 breaths then 10 compressions. Do not do any compressions if there is a pulse, no matter how faint.

(3) Check for a pulse and breathing every 2 minutes. If there is no pulse and breathing, continue for up to 10 minutes before giving up.

ADMINISTERING MEDICINES

As a dog ages, the need to medicate the pet may become more frequent. The ease of giving medicines to dogs may be dependent upon many factors, including the general nature of the dog. Dogs that are aggressive, sensitive, or untrusting may be difficult to treat. The dog's health status also plays a role in the ease of treatment. A dog that feels ill or has a sore mouth or throat might not willingly take oral medication. The past experiences of a dog with medicines and the skill of the person giving the medicines may also affect the pet's attitude about taking pills. Bitter medicines that are inappropriately administered can leave a lasting impression. If your dog objects to the taste, many medicines can be compounded by a pharmacist to have a beef, chicken or fish taste. Ask your veterinarian.

By using the following basic guidelines, medicating your dog may become more efficient and less stressful.

I.   General Rules

A.   Use all medications as prescribed by a veterinarian.

B.   If you do not understand the instructions on the medicine container, contact your veterinarian.

C.   Do not deviate from the dosage or the time interval on the label.

D.   Use all antibiotics until they are gone, unless your veterinarian directs otherwise. Sporadic use of antibiotics can cause bacteria to become resistant to treatment.

E.   Do not give medicine by mouth if your dog is vomiting.

F.   Unless directed by your veterinarian, do not mix medicines in food; your dog may refuse to eat or may not get all of its medicine.

G.   Take your dog's temperature daily to monitor progress. See pages 179-180.

II. Materials Needed
A. Medication(s)
B. Low-fat/low-sodium cheese, bread, or turkey franks
C. Dosage syringe or eye dropper

III. Giving Tablets
A. Option #1 (see illustration below)
   1. Place one hand on the top jaw (maxilla) and one hand on the bottom jaw (mandible).
   2. Tilt your dog's head back.
   3. Open your dog's mouth by applying gentle but firm pressure.
   4. Drop the tablet between the top and bottom sets of canine teeth, aiming for the base of the tongue.
   5. Allow your dog to close its mouth. Watch for your dog to swallow by noting if your dog licks its lips. If your dog spits out the medicine, repeat steps 1-5 or move on to option #2.

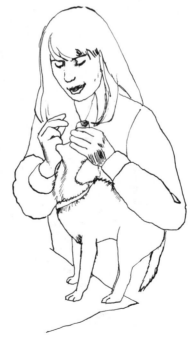

183

B. Option #2
1. With the approval of your veterinarian, choose either low-fat/low-sodium cheese, bread, or turkey franks to wrap the pill inside.
2. Use only tiny portions of food to conceal the pill. You may wish to give one small token piece without a pill prior to giving the portion with the pill to decrease your dog's suspicions. Give the medicine as you would a treat.

C. Option #3
1. Use a combination of the above options 1&2.
2. Use a food to wrap the pill inside, but make sure it is a small piece of food that can be swallowed easily.
3. Follow instructions 1-5 of Option #1.

IV. Giving Liquid Medicine (see illustration below)

A. Fill the eyedropper or dosage syringe with the desired amount of medicine.

B. Insert the eyedropper between the teeth along the side of the mouth by pulling back the lips, or insert the dropper along the side of the mouth in the pocket at the far edge of the lip.

C. Squirt the medicine into your dog's mouth, but be careful not to administer it so fast that it causes your dog to choke.

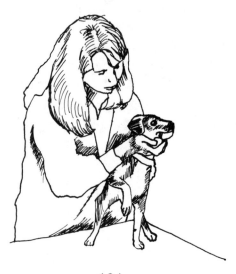

V. Applying Topical Medicine to the Skin

A. Apply the ointment, liquid or spray to the affected area.

B. To prevent the dog from licking off the medicine, involve the dog in an activity to keep its mind off the spot(s) or apply an Elizabethan safety collar (see pages 239-240) if recommended by your veterinarian.

VI. Applying Topical Medicine to the Eye(s)

A. Apply the ointment or drops to the affected eye(s) by approaching your dog from behind and resting your hand on your dog's forehead.

B. Without touching the applicator to the eye, apply the recommended amount of medicine in the eye.

C. Prevent your dog from rubbing its eyes afterward by holding your dog or distracting it with other activities.

VII. Applying Topical Medicine to the Ear(s)

A. Apply the ointment or drops to the affected ear(s) by approaching your dog from behind. Lift the ear flap and clean any debris from the ear canal using a cotton ball (and cleanser if prescribed by your veterinarian).

B. Insert the tip of the container gently into your dog's ear canal and apply the desired amount of medicine into the ear.

C. You may wish to gently massage the ear to distribute the medicine deeper into the ear.

D. If your dog shakes its head violently, hold the dog or distract the pet with other activities. Violent head shaking is a sign of pain, and you should report it to your veterinarian.

ADMINISTERING SUBCUTANEOUS FLUIDS (FLUIDS UNDER THE SKIN)

Some older dogs with health problems may benefit from the administration of fluids under the skin to prevent dehydration and to help dilute internal poisons. The ease of giving these fluids may be dependent upon many factors, such as the general nature of your dog, its health status, past experiences of your dog with medicines, and your skill in giving the fluids. Most dogs tolerate this technique well, especially if the person giving the fluids has had proper instruction and training from a veterinarian. By following the basic guidelines below, giving subcutaneous fluids to your dog may be less stressful. Note that if your dog requires restraint for this procedure, then you will need an assistant (one person to restrain your dog while the other person administers the subcutaneous fluids).

I. General Rules
A. Use subcutaneous fluids only if prescribed by your veterinarian.
B. If you do not understand the instructions for giving the subcutaneous fluids, contact your veterinarian.
C. Do not deviate from the fluid dosage.
D. Stop the use of the fluids if your dog shows signs of pain or becomes combative during treatment. Contact your veterinarian.

II. Materials Needed
A. Sterile needles (usually 18 gauge size)
B. Sterile IV connection tubing
C. Sterile fluids (usually lactated Ringer's solution or saline; the fluids should NOT contain dextrose)

III. Preparing the Fluids

A. Remove the fluid bag from its storage container.

B. Remove the connection tubing from its container, and uncoil it.

C. Remove the plastic plug from the base of the fluid bag.

D. Remove the protective plastic tip from the pointed end of the viewing receptacle/chamber.

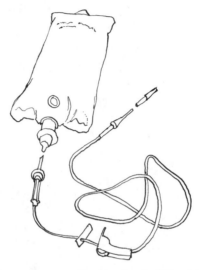

E. Turn the fluid regulator roller to the "off" position to close off the fluids.

F. Insert the pointed end of the connection tube into the base of the bag where the plastic plug was removed. Shove the tip in high enough to break the seal.

G. Hang this unit on a hook at least 2 feet above the dog. (See illustration on page 188.)

H. Squeeze the receptacle chamber so that the chamber fills halfway with fluids.

I. Open the fluid regulator roller to the "on" position. When the fluid fills the entire length of the tubing and dribbles from the end, move the roller to the "off" position.

J. Uncap the hub of the needle, and remove the protective cap from the bottom of the tubing, being careful not to touch either end (to keep them sterile). Place the needle on the bottom of the connective tubing. The fluids are now ready.

187

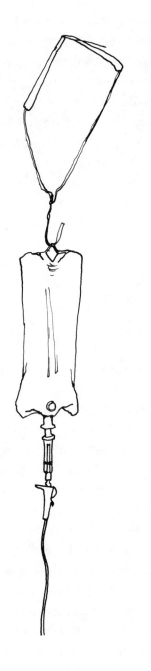

IV. Restraining a Dog to Administer Subcutaneous Fluids

A. Some dogs will allow you to administer subcutaneous fluids without them having to be restrained. If your dog requires restraint for the process of administering subcutaneous fluids, then you will need someone to help (i.e., one person to restrain the dog, and the other to administer the fluids). If restraint is necessary, proceed to step B.

B. Older dogs become confused easier. Be patient and gentle.

C. Arthritis may make regular restraint painful. Again, be gentle.

D. Avoid holding your dog too tightly. Excessive pressure on your dog's chest can interfere with its breathing.

E. Do not forcefully restrain or pull on the legs of an older dog because the bones may fracture easily.

F. Place one arm under your dog's stomach (below the ribs) and the other hand under your dog's neck (with your dog's neck in the corner formed by your elbow). See the illustration on page 160.

V. Giving Subcutaneous Fluids

A. Remove the cap from the needle. Hold the base of the needle (being careful not to touch any other part of the needle) in your right hand.

B. Gently pull up on the loose skin over your dog's shoulder area with your left hand, if you are right handed (or right hand if you are left handed). See the illustration at the top of page 190.

C. Insert the needle under the skin at a 45 degree angle to the skin fold. See the illustration at the bottom of page 190.

D. Let go of the skin you have been holding with your left hand and roll the fluid regulator to the full open position. The fluids should drip quickly or appear as a continuous stream in the receptacle at the top of the connection tubing. If the fluids do not flow freely, turn off the fluids by rolling the fluid regulator to the "off" position. Remove the needle from your dog, and repeat step B and C.

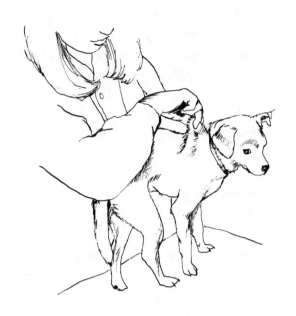

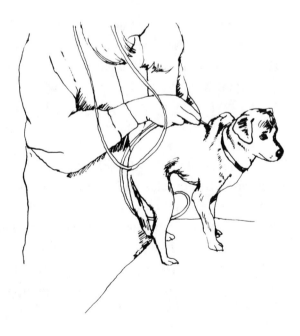

E. When the desired amount has been administered, stop the fluids by rolling the fluid regulator to the "off" position. Each number represents 100 ml of fluids.

F. Remove the needle from under the skin and carefully recap it by scooping up the cap from off the table, so as not to risk sticking your fingers. The needle should be disposed of by your veterinarian. Remove the needle from the connection tubing and replace it with a fresh one for the next treatment.

G. It is common for some fluid to leak out of the skin over the injection site. The loss of fluid can be slowed by applying pressure to the area for 5 minutes, using a clean towel.

HOME DENTAL CARE

Home dental care for your dog may help decrease its risk of developing serious dental problems and decrease the need for involved dental procedures. Remember, proper dental care is one of the simple ways you might help your dog live longer and happier.

One of the most important aspects of developing a dental care plan is to take into account your dog's attitude. Some dogs will allow their owner to handle them in any way, ranging from cleaning their ears to performing toenail trims. Other dogs will not even tolerate having their hair brushed. If you believe that your dog may bite, do not attempt dental care at home.

An older dog that has never had its mouth manipulated can be trained the same way you would train a puppy. First, start by rubbing your dog's face, working your way toward its mouth. You should praise your dog for holding still while you are doing this. Repeat this procedure several times each day until your dog is used to it and does not pull away. Next, while rubbing your dog's mouth, focus on touching and gently lifting the lips. Praise your dog for holding still, and repeat this technique several times a day. Once your dog is used to having its mouth rubbed, show the dog the toothbrush or applicator for applying the dental care product, and rub it on the outside of your dog's mouth. Repeat this until your dog is comfortable with the object being around its mouth. The next step involves lifting the lips and touching the toothbrush or applicator to the teeth and gums. As before, repeat this until your dog is comfortable with it. When your dog readily accepts these procedures, a small portion of hygiene paste, solution or gel may be used. Increase the portion of paste, solution, or gel once your dog is comfortable with the original volume. Depending upon your dog, perfecting these exercises may take several minutes to several days. For the best results, dental hygiene should be practiced every day.

There are many dental products available for dogs. Besides a variety of pastes, sprays, solutions and gels, there are enzyme-coated rawhide chews and dental exercise toys. The pastes, sprays, solutions, and gels are designed to be applied to the teeth by using a pet toothbrush or a child's toothbrush, finger toothbrush, gauze sponge, or cotton applicator. The pastes are probably the most palatable; they come in a variety of flavors, including malt and poultry flavors.

Never use human pastes because they foam too much, and the foaming is offensive to most dogs. Also, human toothpaste may make your dog ill if your dog ingests it.

For dogs that resist teeth cleaning, there are still good options for proper dental hygiene. The rawhide chews with enzymes allow your dog to do the work. When your dog chews on these, its mouth is exposed to the enzymes, and plaque is broken down. Another option is dental care toys that can be filled with dog toothpaste; when your dog chews on one of these toys, the paste is released onto its teeth. Ask your veterinarian for advice regarding which method is most appropriate for your dog.

When performing dental hygiene, make sure you treat all of the teeth, but concentrate on those that are prone to getting the most buildup. When brushing or wiping solutions onto the teeth, brush or wipe away from the gum line. If the gums bleed after home dental care, consult your veterinarian before continuing.

To treat the teeth on the inside of the mouth near the tongue, use a Nylabone® as a wedge in the mouth (i.e., place the Nylabone® sideways in the mouth so that it is sticking out of the mouth on both sides, and then hold the mouth shut). This technique will enable you to clean the insides of the teeth safely. Do not use any object as a wedge that might hurt your dog's teeth or anything that might break from the pressure of your dog's bite. Note that not all dogs will tolerate this procedure, but fortunately the inside of the teeth are usually less affected by plaque.

There are many signs of dental disease that are cause for concern and should be reported promptly to a veterinarian. They include reddened or bleeding gums, calculus (tartar) buildup on a tooth, pus around a tooth, sore gums, bad breath, a lump or bump in the mouth, and any loose teeth.

The following basic guidelines are a summary of the information presented above. By following these guidelines, you should be better able to promote good dental hygiene for your dog at home.

Special Considerations for Dental Care of Older Dogs

A. Choose a paste, solution or spray, or gel recommended by your veterinarian.

B. Choose a child's toothbrush, pet toothbrush, finger toothbrush, gauze sponge, or cotton-tipped applicator.

C. Gradually accustom your dog to having its mouth handled, and then slowly introduce the toothbrush or other cleaning device to your dog. Once your dog is used to the toothbrush or cleaning device, apply small quantities of the paste or other cleaning agent to its teeth.

D. If your dog will not tolerate having its mouth handled, choose enzyme-covered rawhide chews, dental exerciser toys, and/or a hygiene solution mixed into the pet's drinking water as a substitute for brushing.

E. Use products daily.

F. Report any problems to your veterinarian, including reddened or bleeding gums, calculus (tartar) buildup on the teeth, pus around a tooth, sore gums, bad breath, a lump or bump in the mouth, or any loose teeth.

G. If the gums bleed after dental care, consult your veterinarian before continuing.

PART 5

TREATMENT OPTIONS

INTRODUCTORY INFORMATION

For most aging dogs with medical problems, there are several treatment options. Hospitalization, outpatient treatment, alternative treatments (e.g., acupuncture), house calls and pet hospice may all be viable options. The option(s) that you choose should be based on your dog's needs and personality, as well as the resources that are available.

Your veterinarian will give you information and options, but ultimately many tough decisions will be yours to make. At times, you may wish to seek a second opinion from another veterinarian, especially if the situation calls for a specialist, but still you will have to decide the best course of treatment for your pet. The following pages will help acquaint you with the different types of treatment options and give you a better understanding of how to make the most of the option(s) you select. You will learn the questions you should ask yourself and your veterinarian regarding your possible choices, and you will learn how to use the answers to make the best possible decisions.

HOSPITALIZATION

Hospitalization may be an option for a dog that is ill or injured. Hospitalization should be considered under a variety of circumstances: (1) when a dog requires treatment that cannot be practically administered at home, (2) when a dog cannot take its medicine by mouth, (3) when constant skilled observation or monitoring is required, or (4) for recovery from surgery.

Some dogs exhibit high levels of fright or stress while being away from home, and they might not benefit as much from hospitalization as dogs that are less stressed. If your dog exhibits high stress or fear when away from home, discuss other options with your veterinarian. If other options fall short of the care the dog needs, hospitalization may still be best. Refer to the the other sections for other options for treatment.

When your pet is ill, you should make a list of questions for your veterinarian. In this chapter, a list of questions has been compiled for you, although you may wish to add more, depending upon the situation. If your dog does need hospitalization, don't simply ask the questions; also write down the answers. If you make a written record of the answers, you will be better able to track your dog's progress based on the initial observations of the veterinarian.

I. **Basic Guidelines**

A. Provide the veterinarian in charge with a telephone number where someone can be reached at all times so that any changes in your dog's condition or treatment can be discussed.

B. Check with the veterinarian or hospital staff regarding their pet visitation policy. Visitation is helpful not only for your pet but also for you.

C. If financial constraints are affecting the care your dog may receive, inquire whether financial aid is available.

D. Determine how many progress reports will be shared during the day and whether you should call the veterinary staff or they should call you.

197

II. Questions To Ask About the Problem

A. What is my dog's problem?

B. Does my pet have more than one problem, and, if so, are the problems related?

C. If there are several possible problems, are there tests to confirm the diagnosis?

III. Questions to Ask About Determining the Problem (Diagnosis)

A. What tests are available to diagnose my pet's problem?

B. What information will the tests provide?

C. Can the test results change the type of treatment my dog is receiving?

D. What is the cost of testing?

E. How invasive are the tests? How much pain will they cause and is there any risk associated with the tests?

IV. Questions To Ask About the Outcome (Prognosis)

A. What can I expect my dog's future to be like?

B. Will this condition return?

C. Will this condition have any long-term side effects?

D. What is an average recovery time?

V. Questions To Ask About the Treatment

A. What will the treatment involve?

B. How much time will treatments take?

C. How expensive are the medications?

D. What side effects will be involved with the medicines?

E. If surgery is recommended:

(1) Is there more than one procedure that can be done?

(2) Is there a medical alternative to a surgical procedure?

(3) How many of these surgeries do you perform per year? (The more surgeries, the better.)

(4) Should I see a specialist?

F. What type of care will need to be provided after my dog returns home?

G. Are follow-up veterinary visits recommended?

OUTPATIENT TREATMENT

Outpatient treatment is an alternative for dogs who do not need hospitalization, cannot cope with hospitalization, or whose owners cannot or choose not to afford hospitalization. This option may be recommended for dogs that do not cope well being away from home; the added stress of being in a hospital may hinder the recovery period for a highly anxious or stressed dog. Some dogs that are stressed from being away from home do not eat well and do not get the necessary rest for a good recovery. Outpatient treatment is not recommended for dogs that are continually vomiting and cannot keep medicine or food down. Nor is outpatient treatment recommended in any situation that requires constant monitoring or supervision. One benefit of hospitalization is that it can be a highly controlled environment with immediate emergency medical resources and personnel available to address any urgent needs.

If your dog does not cope well with being in a veterinary hospital, discuss the situation with your veterinarian and determine the relative merits and disadvantages of outpatient versus inpatient treatment. Frequently, the situation does not have a clear-cut answer, and the best course of action is a matter of good judgment by you and your veterinarian. Sometimes a doctor may recommend twenty-four hours of outpatient treatment and then reassess the condition. Regardless of whether the initial decision is for inpatient or outpatient care, your dog's response to treatment will dictate whether any changes are advisable.

Outpatient treatment may involve giving your dog various medicines by mouth and/or feeding your dog special foods. Your abilities to assist your dog, and control its environment in a constructive manner will dictate your effectiveness with follow-up care at home. If your dog is seen on an outpatient basis for a medical problem, you should monitor your dog closely at home and take note of its food and water intake, bowel movements and urinations, and any behavioral changes or signs of illness.

ACUPUNCTURE

Acupuncture is a technique that is now finding its time and place in the treatment of animals. Acupuncture can be used on animals to lessen and alleviate pain and to treat disease. It is a method of treatment that can provide a more holistic approach to a medical problem.

Some general guidelines, combined with the advice of your veterinarian, will help you decide if acupuncture may help your dog. First, note that the timing of acupuncture is critical. Acupuncture should not begin prior to an accurate diagnosis because acupuncture can change the signs the dog is showing, thereby making diagnosis more difficult. Delay in diagnosis of certain problems could be life threatening.

There are precautions to follow just prior to acupuncture. Dogs should not undergo acupuncture if they have just eaten a large meal, are frightened or anxious, are pregnant, or have just been bathed. Certain medications may interfere with treatment, and you should therefore remind your veterinarian about any medications your dog is taking.

The technique of acupuncture involves stimulating points throughout the body to release pain-blocking chemicals from the brain (called beta-endorphins) or by changing the nervous system to alter blood pressure, digestion, and the release of other body chemicals. The points can be stimulated in a variety of ways, ranging from applying pressure to the areas (via the acupuncturist's fingers), inserting needles, applying a type of vacuum over the area, changing the temperature over the area, or injecting areas with compounds such as saline or vitamins. Ultrasound, implants, electronic devices, and lasers can also be used to stimulate these areas. The acceptance and usefulness of each technique varies.

Treatment schedules vary according to the ailment, but in general, with sudden problems, the more frequent the treatment, the faster the relief. Generally, the longer the treatment continues, the better the pain relief, and the longer the effects. Depending upon the circumstances, treatments may need to be repeated every 2-3 days for several weeks.

Note that it is illegal for a person without a veterinary degree to practice acupuncture on an animal without the supervision of a veterinarian. Stimulation of the wrong areas, insertion of needles into vital organs, and not recognizing the contraindications before acupuncture can result in great risk to the dog. Make sure you choose a veterinarian who has been well trained in the technique. If your veterinarian does not perform acupuncture and you are interested in this option, consult with your veterinarian about finding a reputable acupuncturist. Also discuss with your veterinarian the relative usefulness of acupuncture techniques for your dog's situation, and make sure you keep your original veterinarian informed of the decisions, treatments, and progress if you proceed with another veterinarian.

HOUSE CALLS

If the stress of your dog's medical problem is distracting you from other matters in your life and you feel your dog needs more attention, then house calls may be an ideal solution. House calls are an important part of veterinary medicine, but unfortunately many veterinarians do not offer this service. In addition to the fact that some dogs are better treated in their home environment, there are some owners who are unable to travel to a veterinarian. In general, most dogs are more relaxed in their own environment; however, some become very territorial toward an unfamiliar guest, especially if the guest smells like a veterinarian. Use your best judgment to decide whether house calls are best for you and your pet.

Most cities have veterinarians who make house calls on a full or part-time basis. If you do not have a recommendation for a house-call veterinarian, you might find one in the Yellow Pages of your phone book. If you live in a community where no house-call service is listed, your veterinarian might make a house call if time permits; you have nothing to lose by asking.

The services that can be provided at the house vary according to the veterinarian's set up. Some house call veterinarians drive fully-equipped mobile hospitals and can perform surgery and X-rays at the home. Other veterinarians may bring only necessary medications but may still have the capabilities to run blood tests and perform ECG's and minor procedures. Regardless of the services offered, you must make sure you are comfortable with your selection of a house-call veterinarian. See pages 22-23 for finding a veterinarian.

If house calls are not available in your area and transportation to the veterinary hospital is a problem, there may be a pet taxi service available. Your veterinarian may recommend one, or else you might find one in the Yellow Pages phone directory.

Another situation in which house calls may offer an advantage is if your dog needs to be euthanized. You and your dog may be more comfortable being in familiar surroundings. See Part 7 of this book starting on page 215 regarding this difficult decision.

WHEN TO GET A SECOND OPINION

There may be a time in your dog's life when you want to get a second opinion regarding medical care. Under most circumstances, a dog's regular veterinarian should be receptive to the idea of getting a second opinion, because another professional opinion will ensure proper diagnosis and provide confidence about the medical decisions that are made. Most veterinarians encourage second opinions if there is more information needed to make a definitive diagnosis or to select the best treatment.

The most obvious circumstance in which a second opinion is warranted is when your veterinarian recommends an opinion by a specialist. Often this will occur when more specialized treatment is appropriate. Because veterinary medicine is highly complex, some veterinarians spend additional years training in particular areas of specialty, in the same manner that some medical doctors specialize in particular areas of human medicine. For example, a dog that has congestive heart failure may benefit from being referred to a cardiologist (i.e., a heart specialist).

Another circumstance in which a second opinion is warranted may be when major surgery is required for your dog. If time permits and there is any question about the necessity of surgery, definitely get a second opinion. In certain circumstances, there may be medical alternatives that avoid or postpone surgery. For example, bladder stones that can be treated by surgery might also be treated by a special diet to dissolve the stones. (Unfortunately, not all dogs respond to the special diet.) Bladder stones might also be removed by cystoscopy (removal of the stones via a special fiberoptic scope). Also, if your dog has a problem that is difficult to diagnose, sometimes a fresh outlook or opinion from a specialist is advisable, especially if most diagnostic resources have been exhausted.

A second opinion may also be warranted if your dog is not responding to treatment after the therapy has been given a chance to work. (It is important, though, in this circumstance, that you have administered the treatments correctly and on a timely basis. Then, if your dog has not responded, talk with your veterinarian to determine

203

whether an adjustment in the treatment might solve the problem.)

Another time a second opinion may be warranted is when you feel something is not right with the situation. It is important that you are comfortable with your decisions and with the treatment that is taking place, and if you are not, then you should talk with another veterinarian. The question lists provided on pages 22-23 and on page 198 may help you obtain the information you need to make the best decisions.

DECISION-MAKING WORKSHEET

In previous chapters we have discussed various options that may be available regarding places and methods of medical treatment for your dog. In many situations involving medical treatment for your dog, trying to make a decision can be confusing. The worksheet that follows has been designed to provide a set of questions to establish what is important for you and your dog. Answer these questions to help determine your best options.

I. Questions to Ask Yourself

A. Is my dog uncomfortable away from home?

B. Am I able to give prescribed medicines at home?

C. Is my dog able to take medicine by mouth? If not, is the problem that my dog vomits the medicine, or is the medicine too difficult to administer?

D. Can my dog get up and go outside? If not, am I able to carry the pet?

E. Is my dog able to eat? If so, how much, and does the food stay down?

F. Is my dog able to control its urinations?

G. Is my dog able to control its bowel movements?

H. Can I provide the nursing care my dog requires?

II. Questions to Ask the Doctor

A. What is the recommended treatment?

B. If it were your dog, what treatment would you choose?

C. What is the difference in the costs of the different possibilities?

D. If my dog is hospitalized, may I visit?

E. What is my dog's chance of recovery? Will one type of treatment give a faster recovery rate than another?

F.   What is the estimated recovery time?

G.   When do I need to make a decision?

III. How to Interpret the Answers

A.   If you answered "no" to any question in Part I Questions B through H above, consider hospitalization as an option. Consider your response to Part I Question A (Is my dog uncomfortable away from home?) in making the decision.

B.   Consult with your veterinarian regarding the questions in Part II.

C.   If your decision is influenced by financial constraints, consult with your veterinarian about financial options that might be available.

D.   Discuss the situation with family members.

E.   If a decision does not need to be made immediately, take the time you need to make the decision that is right for you and your pet.

PART 6

—

ANESTHESIA AND SURGERY

MINIMIZING RISKS

Often as a dog ages there will come a time when surgery or anesthesia may be required. The decision of consenting to a procedure may be worrisome because of the increased risk of anesthesia associated with an older dog. Regardless of age, there is always some risk associated with anesthetics, but modern advances in veterinary medicine have decreased the risks compared to fifteen years ago. Specifically, advances in new anesthetics and monitoring equipment have helped with safety.

Most veterinarians take many precautions prior to, during, and after general anesthesia and surgery to minimize the risk to your dog. A complete health checkup is crucial prior to any procedure involving general anesthesia or surgery. The health check should start with an examination of your dog's eyes, ears, mouth, heart, lungs, abdomen, skin, reflexes, temperature, and rectum. Next, especially in older dogs, your veterinarian should perform tests on your dog's stool (i.e., a fecal examination), urine (i.e., a urinalysis), and blood (i.e., a blood profile, complete blood count and possibly a thyroid analysis).

The fecal examination is used to detect parasites that may compromise your dog's health and pose an anesthetic risk. The stool specimen is examined with a microscope to check for parasites that cannot always be seen by the naked eye. The stool is also examined for blood and mucus. The urinalysis is used to obtain information on kidney and liver functions, plus it can screen for diabetes and hormonal diseases and urinary tract infections.

The blood profile, which is actually a series of five to fifteen different tests, also yields a wide range of information. It is one of the best tests to screen for changes occurring in your dog's organs. Blood profile tests require only a small amount of blood, yet they may uncover hidden changes in the liver, kidneys, bones, and pancreas. The blood profile also measures the levels of electrolytes, such as sodium, potassium, and phosphorus, and thereby serves to alert the veterinarian to the possible presence of a variety of disease conditions. The blood profile includes a measurement of the protein levels, which may point to certain cancers or other metabolic problems, and it includes a blood sugar level test which checks for diabetes.

208

Another blood test called a complete blood count is commonly used to screen for disease. It gives information about the presence of infection, inflammation, blood cancers, anemias, and dehydration by examining the red blood cells and white blood cells in the body. It also checks the platelet count, which is important in clotting.

In addition to the blood profile and the complete blood count, your veterinarian may wish to perform a thyroid analysis. This test typically checks for a thyroid deficiency by measuring the amount of thyroid hormone in the blood. The test is warranted when a dog shows signs of a thyroid deficiency, such as weight gain, hair loss, lethargy, and/or having chills.

The presurgery, and ideally preanesthesia, health checkup should also include radiographs (i.e., X-rays) to screen for aging changes or to further investigate a potential problem. Radiographs are an affordable noninvasive way to look inside a dog to evaluate the size, shape, and position of various organs. Radiographs can also uncover the presence of fluids, stones, foreign objects, and/or air in inappropriate places. Radiographs are especially important prior to anesthesia and surgery because they are used to evaluate the dog's heart size and to check to make sure that the dog's lungs are clear.

Finally, your dog's health examination prior to receiving general anesthesia or undergoing surgery should include an ECG (also called an EKG or electrocardiogram). The ECG is a test that measures electrical changes in the heart, including changes that can disrupt the functioning of the heart. It can discover abnormal rhythms (arrhythmias) of the heart, and it can indirectly confirm heart enlargement as well as give some indication of the seriousness of any heart condition. Some changes in the ECG may also be suggestive of electrolyte imbalances, fluid around the heart, and shock. The ECG is a noninvasive test that is very useful both prior to and during surgery.

After your dog has received a complete health checkup, your veterinarian should inform you of the relative risks of general anesthesia and surgery versus other treatments, or no treatments, based on the tests that were performed. If you and your veterinarian decide to proceed with the general anesthesia and/or surgery, your veterinarian will use a variety of monitoring devices during the anesthesia or surgical procedure to minimize the risk. Most veterinarians will have a registered veterinary technician monitor your dog's anesthesia closely. The technician, along with the veterinarian, is responsible for watching the depth of the anesthesia by monitoring your dog's pulse rate and strength, respiratory rate and depth, eye reflex, and jaw tone. Extra safety is achieved by also using monitoring equipment. A respiratory monitor is used to check the rate of breathing; if your dog stops breathing for a designated period of time (e.g., twenty seconds) an alarm will sound alerting the technician and veterinarian to breathe for the dog (i.e., pump oxygen into your dog's lungs). A pulse oximeter is another piece of safety equipment used by veterinarians to minimize the risk of anesthesia. It is used to monitor the amount of oxygen in a dog's blood and to monitor the pulse rate. The pulse oximeter also is equipped with an alarm system to alert the veterinarian early when a problem begins to develop. An ECG (discussed above) can also be used to monitor changes of the heart function during surgery. Other means of monitoring include a pulse amplifier, to enable the veterinarian to actually hear the dog's pulse, and an esophageal stethoscope, which is placed down the throat over the area where the heart is located in order to hear the heartbeat better. Finally, your veterinarian will monitor blood pressure by using an ultrasonic doppler device or an oscillometric cuff.

After care is an important aspect for recovery from general anesthesia and surgery. Proper monitoring during the wake-up period is as important as during the procedure. Some life-threatening complications can occur after anesthesia, including the aspiration of vomitus, hypothermia (becoming chilled), hyperthermia (becoming overheated) and post-operative hemorrhage (i.e., bleeding). Complications that are discovered early have the best chance for good results. Note that some dogs benefit from certain medicines that can be administered prior to general anesthesia to avoid complications. Consult your veterinarian.

ELECTIVE VERSUS URGENT PROCEDURES

The decision to perform surgery may depend upon the urgency, the benefits, the risks, and the costs of the procedure. Emergencies, for example a dog that has a ruptured spleen, may require immediate surgery to remedy a life-threatening situation. In that case, the decision to enter into surgery may be an easy one, if the cost of the procedure is within your financial means. If the procedure is one that has many benefits for the animal's comfort and few risks, the advantages help justify the procedure. For example, if your otherwise healthy ten-year-old dog has severe dental disease that causes your dog great pain and has an immediate risk of spreading infection from the mouth to critical organs, the benefits outweigh the risks of the anesthetic. Your veterinarian can help educate you about the urgency, benefits, risks, and costs of treatment options and help guide you in making difficult decisions regarding your pet.

Some common elective procedures for older dogs include dentistries, removal of cysts, ear cleaning, ovariohysterectomies (spaying) and orchiectomies (neutering). Many of these cases are considered elective; however, there are special circumstances under which procedures that are typically elective can become urgent. Your veterinarian should be able to advise you appropriately.

Urgent procedures include clearing a urinary blockage, removing a diseased organ, such as the spleen, removing an abscess (pocket of infection), closing lacerations, treating fractures, removing tumors, and anything else where time is of the essence in protecting the health of your pet. Your veterinarian will tell you whether a situation is urgent.

In older dogs, procedures that are elective should be considered because they may be crucial for the long-term health and well-being of the pet. Dental procedures are one such example. Often a pet is better off in the long run having elective dental procedures rather than waiting until the situation requires action. Ask your veterinarian about the long-term consequences of a decision for or against elective procedures, and ask about the window of opportunity for a procedure; depending upon your dog's age and condition, anesthesia and/or surgery may be an appropriate option now, but not later.

Depending upon your dog's condition and the relative urgency of the situation, your veterinarian may advise delaying a procedure in order to better prepare your dog for the event. For example, your veterinarian may feel a need to better stabilize your dog's condition prior to surgery via the use of medications and/or fluids. Additionally, if your dog is overweight, your veterinarian may recommend weight loss prior to an elective procedure.

LASER SURGERY

Laser surgery has replaced traditional surgery as the treatment of choice for a wide variety of procedures. Anytime your pet needs surgery, inquire about the relative benefits of laser surgery for your dog's particular circumstances.

Because our older dogs sometimes have slower recoveries after surgery compared to younger pets, it is in their best interest to minimize the invasiveness of any necessary procedures. The laser is a precise tool which uses highly focused light particles to cut tissues. Unlike conventional surgery tools, the laser has the ability to seal tissues as it cuts. When a laser cuts nerve endings, the nerves are sealed in a way that dramatically reduces pain sensations. By sealing blood vessels, the laser reduces the amount of blood loss for the pet. Laser surgery also seals lymph vessels and thereby helps prevent swelling. (Lymph vessels carry lymph, a substance which bathes the body's organs.) Though healing time is not always reduced by using a laser to perform surgery, the decreased pain, decreased blood loss and decreased swelling generally make the dog feel substantially better after the procedure than would be expected with traditional surgery.

The laser has opened new treatment options for older dogs. Small skin lumps and bumps can often be removed without the use of a general anesthetic. Eye surgery, mouth surgery, and surgery for lick granulomas (nonhealing sores) are examples of situations where use of a laser typically offers a safer procedure with fewer complications than traditional surgery. In fact, many types of surgery can be performed better with the use of a laser. Ask your veterinarian about the availability, relative benefits and cost of laser surgery for your pet. Older dogs tend to have a more difficult recovery period than younger dogs, and laser surgery may provide the extra benefit that your dog needs.

ENDOSCOPIC PROCEDURES

Endoscopy is a procedure that uses a special optic instrument, called an endoscope, for examination inside a pet's body. Veterinarians use this tool to gather important information about your pet's health that other tests cannot provide. Endoscopy may be warranted any time your pet experiences a medical condition that your veterinarian is unable to diagnose and/or treat in a routine manner. Any time your veterinarian suggests that exploratory surgery may be necessary for your pet, you should inquire about endoscopy options. Endoscopy is often performed by a specialist; ask whether your veterinarian performs endoscopic procedures, and if not, ask for a referral to a specialist who does.

Endoscopy allows your pet's doctor to look at internal structures to make sure they are the correct size, shape, and color. The procedure can also allow your doctor to observe the internal function of some organs. With endoscopy, your veterinarian can see internal foreign objects, ulcers, inflamed areas (e.g., stomach, bowels, sinuses, bladder, pancreas, heart, joints), polyps, tumors (benign and malignant), strictures (narrowing) and obstructions, infections, tendon and ligament ruptures, collapsed trachea or lungs, enlarged organs, and a host of other problems and disease conditions.

The procedure may be used not only to diagnose, but also to treat your pet, depending upon the problem. For example, endoscopy can be used to remove a foreign object from the digestive tract or remove stones from the bladder. Also, it may be used to collect difficult-to-reach diagnostic specimens. Endoscopy is also useful for tracking the progress of recovery and alerting the doctor if therapy needs to be changed.

There are different types and sizes of scopes to examine different areas of the pet's body. Your veterinarian will choose which procedure and equipment type is best for your pet. Most endoscopic procedures require that your pet be under a general anesthetic. However, unlike more invasive surgical procedures that require long recovery times, most endoscopy procedures are done on an outpatient basis. Your veterinarian will discuss details of your pet's situation and expected recovery.

PART 7

—

FINAL DECISIONS AND
COPING WITH LOSS

GENERAL INFORMATION

As a dog owner, perhaps the most stressful experience you will ever encounter begins when your pet approaches the end of its natural lifespan or when a terminal condition is drawing to a close. It is sometimes during that difficult time that we come to realize the great importance our pet has played in our life. Reflecting on the joys and impending sorrow may seem more bitter than sweet, but with time, and perhaps with the aid of this chapter of this book, you will come to a time and place where your reflections evoke mostly positive feelings. This chapter is as much for you as it is for your pet, because your pet's final days are a journey for you both.

In the past several years, there has been a growing awareness of the magnitude of loss and the emotional turmoil associated with the passing of a pet. This chapter is designed to lay the groundwork to help you through an emotionally difficult time and to aid in making difficult decisions during your pet's final days with you. You will learn that you have many options and many responsibilities, and you will find that by taking a proactive stance in dealing with this difficult situation, you will help yourself and your pet through the process.

If you are reading this book for the first time, and this situation does not yet apply to you, make a mental note now to reread these pages when the time does come.

PET HOSPICE

Pet hospice is a service provided by some veterinary hospitals. It consists of home and hospital care for terminally ill patients. Hospice care continues to evolve to meet more needs of the dog and the family. The idea of pet hospice is that when a dog can no longer benefit from treatment, it is time for the dog to go into hospice care where the pet can be in familiar surroundings near the people who share the pet's love during the final days.

Veterinarians are trained to prevent suffering in dogs with terminal illnesses and to provide quality end-of-life care. In order to accomplish these goals, a combination of methods is employed to provide comprehensive care for your dog. A veterinarian with an understanding of hospice should be able to design a plan for your dog based on your desires and needs. The plan, at a minimum, should include the following:

10 Guidelines for Hospice Care of Dogs
1. Provide comfort with good pain management.
2. Provide clean, soft bedding.
3. Maintain proper thermal comfort by providing warmth or by keeping your dog cool as needed.
4. Prevent dry, sore mouth by use of a mouth moisturizer.
5. Prevent dry, sore eyes by use of an eye lubricant or artificial tears.
6. Provide relief from nausea and breathing difficulties via use of medications.
7. Provide proper nutrition based on your dog's disease.
8. Keep your dog clean and dry by performing proper hygiene. See pages 171-173.
9. Provide frequent opportunities for your dog to urinate and defecate.
10. Provide attention to satisfy your dog's emotional needs, as well as your own.

DESIGNING A SUPPORT SYSTEM

As your dog ages and approaches the end of its lifespan, you should develop a support system to help you cope with the final days and the period immediately thereafter. By organizing a support system in advance, you will have it when you need it. Support and strength can be gathered through friends, family, your church, a pet-loss support group (check, or call, you local newspaper) or a professional grief counselor. Additionally, some people find strength and solace in the pursuit of certain personal activities (e.g., athletic, social, etc.).

Some people do not choose to share their strong feelings about their dog with others, perhaps because of difficulty in expressing the intense bonding between pet and owner, or perhaps because they feel that their experience is an intensely personal feeling, and that they should not violate the privacy of the emotions between themselves and their dog. However, in spite of any natural tendency you may have toward emotional isolation, you should note that sharing the experience with the right person or people can be extremely important emotionally. And while the act of turning to someone for support may be difficult in its first steps, once you begin the process, you will likely be grateful that you made the effort.

The following outline can be used to prepare a means of support, when you need it, to get you through the difficult time associated with the passing of your pet. Use those parts of the outline that seem most appropriate based on your anticipated personal needs.

I.   Support By People

A.   Make a list of all family members who are intimately associated with your dog.

B.   On the same sheet of paper make a list of friends who are intimately associated with your dog.

C.   On a second sheet of paper make a list of family members who would be sympathetic to your feelings about your dog.

D. On the same sheet of paper, make a list of friends who would be sympathetic to your feelings about your dog.

E. List family and friends who you think would not understand your feelings about your dog.

II. Support By Activities

A. Keep a daily diary of your feelings during this time.

B. Record your dog's daily activities.

C. Volunteer time at a local shelter.

D. Write stories about the pets at the shelter.

E. Gather information on pet-loss organizations and hotline numbers. Ask your veterinarian or do a search on the internet.

III. Support By Other Pets

A. Make a list of other pets in the household, past and present.

B. Make a list of other pets belonging to family or friends.

IV. How to Use the Above Information

A. Keep the above information in a folder so that you have access to all of it as needed.

B. Refer to the lists of friends and family who share your sympathies regarding your dog. Share your feelings with the people on that list, and ask them to share their feelings with you. Helping someone else through the difficult period can be extremely beneficial for your own emotional state.

C. Plan activities with family and friends who are sympathetic. Activities with sympathetic family and friends will allow you to have healthy social interactions in the context of a supportive group.

D. Plan activities that include some family and friends who you believe may not understand your feelings. This will enable you to experience social interactions that are separate from anything having to do with your dog, and may help give you a needed, healthy break from your focus on your grief.

E. In addition to writing in your diary, occasionally review the writings in your diary. Often writings that seem awkward or inadequate at the time, seem to have remarkable clarity and insight later.

F. Review the summary of your dog's activities. You may find great satisfaction in knowing that during the last days and weeks you shared quality time with your pet. In the midst of your grief, focus on the quality of what you shared and the fullness of your dog's life.

G. Spend extra time with other pets in the family that might need your attention; they will be there for support when your dog passes away. If you currently have no other pets but had a pet in the past, allow your thoughts to focus on how that pet added to your life. Past pets enable us to know that immediate grief will fade while the joyful memories will remain.

H. Share stories of pets with family and friends. Focusing on the joys of pets may be painful at first, but helpful afterward.

I. Get to know better the pets of friends and family. While the bond that you have with a special pet can never be transferred, that bond should enable you to relate better to other people's pets, and your interaction with those pets can be emotionally satisfying.

J. Consider volunteering time at a local animal shelter. The experience will put you into contact with grateful dogs that need attention, and it will help take your focus temporarily off of you grief because you will be redirecting your emotional energies into a constructive outlet. To make the most of the experience, write about the animals you encounter and how they respond to you.

K. Call a pet loss organization or a pet loss hotline. Having the opportunity to talk with people who are going through a similar pet loss can be incredibly beneficial. Do not underestimate the emotional value of this type of experience.

L. Allow time for the grieving process so that you can better appreciate and take care of a new pet when you are ready.

THE LAST DAYS

The dying process can be a very unsettling event, especially if you do not know what to expect. Understanding the events prior to your pet's passing may help in making the decision to euthanize or to not intervene. In general, there are three scenarios that apply to a pet's death. The dog may die unexpectedly, quickly from a illness, or gradually from a chronic condition. The following generalizations apply to most situations, but not to every individual; not all dogs react the same.

When a dog dies suddenly and unexpected, there is no time for the owner to prepare for the loss. One fortunate aspect of sudden passing is that the dog does not suffer long; however, sometimes there are increased feelings of guilt. These feelings often are the result of the fact that in hindsight, any pet owner would have spent more time with the pet if he or she had known that the pet was living its last days. The guilt can be even greater if the death resulted from an accident. Counseling may be especially helpful in these situations.

When a dog suffers from a sudden illness, there is limited time to prepare for the death, but there are decisions that the owner can make about the course of the dog's last days. Aggressive pet hospice to prevent suffering may be a good option. The more you do for your dog to make the pet comfortable in the final days, the easier your grief process will be; during your grief, you will have the consolation of knowing that you helped your pet as best you could when the pet needed you the most. Your support system may be of help in this situation. (See pages 218-220.)

Chronic illness and certain conditions related to aging may linger for a long time before your pet eventually has its final day. During the prolonged period of time associated with many chronic situations, much preparation can be made. You can make decisions that can affect the comfort of your dog now as well as later, toward the end. The amount of discomfort your dog experiences will vary depending upon the particular circumstances, but your veterinarian will be able to inform you about the situation and provide you with options for your pet. Ask your veterinarian to design a pet hospice program for your dog. Also, note that long illnesses can be both emotionally and physically draining for you, and you may need to use your support system to help you throughout the process.

The time may come when you are faced with the decision of whether to euthanize your pet. This decision can be extremely emotionally difficult. With our pets, we have the ultimate power regarding final decisions: whether to intervene in an attempt to extend life, to intervene to end the suffering, or to not intervene in the life process. Your decision will be one that is personal to you, and the choice that you make will be dictated by both your pet's circumstances and your own personal philosophies. To the extent possible, attempt to make the decision based on what you perceive to be the pet's best interest rather than your own. The final issue you need to consider is whether your pet is ready to die, not whether you are ready for your pet to die. Your veterinarian should be able to help answer questions regarding this issue. Regardless of whether your pet's final day is today or some later day, make sure that your pet is suffering as little as possible. Allow your dog the opportunity to leave this world in as comfortable a manner as possible.

Sometimes doubt about any decision we choose haunts us afterward. Confront your doubts by telling yourself that you made the best decisions you were able to make at the time. Regardless of your decisions, one of the most important things you can do for your dog and yourself is to let your dog know that you are there for him/her and that he/she is loved during those last days or moments. But even if you cannot be with your dog physically at the end, the lifetime of shared love should carry both of you through this difficult time.

WORKSHEET FOR DECISION MAKING

The following worksheet has been designed to help you get the information you need to make the difficult decisions for your dog as the pet approaches the end of its life. Your answers to the questions on this worksheet should serve to help you focus on the immediate relevant issues and thereby reach a decision. You may wish to discuss this worksheet with other family members or with your veterinarian.

I.   Questions to Ask Yourself

A.   Is my dog comfortable?

B.   Am I able to give prescribed medicines at home? Is my dog able to digest the medications, or is my dog vomiting after I administer the medications?

C.   Are the medicines helping?

D.   Can my dog get up to go out to the bathroom? If not, am I able to carry my dog?

E.   Is my dog able to eat? If so, how much and does it stay down?

F.   Is my dog able to control its urinations?

G.   Is my dog able to control its bowel movements?

H.   Can I provide the nursing care my dog requires?

I.   If my dog is dying, would I prefer to have my dog at home or in the hospital?

II.   Questions to Ask the Doctor

A.   Does my dog have a terminal condition?

B.   What is the recommended treatment?

C.   If my dog is hospitalized, may I visit with him/her?

D.   What is my dog's chance for recovery? Will one type of treatment give a better chance for recovery or a faster recovery rate than another?

E.   What is the estimated recovery time, or if recovery is not expected, how much time does my pet have left?

F. What type of quality life can I expect for my pet in the time remaining?

G. Is my dog suffering now?

H. Would my dog benefit from hospice care?

III. Dealing with the Answers

A. You, with the help of your veterinarian, are probably the best person to decide what is best for your pet, because most likely you know your pet better than anybody else.

B. Reread the questions and answers as often as necessary to reach your decision. If there are any other questions that you think should be relevant to your decision process, add them to the lists along with their answers.

C. If your decision is influenced by financial constraints, consult with your veterinarian about deferred payment options that might be available.

If your particular situation and your philosophy leads you to consider euthanasia, you may want to consider having it done at your home. Your dog and you may experience more comfort being in familiar surroundings. After the fact, you may find some comfort in knowing that your dog was not stressed with a final trip to the hospital. Most cities have veterinarians who make house calls on a full or part-time basis. If you live in a community where no house call service is listed, you may want to inquire with your veterinarian; some veterinarians will make house calls if time permits or if it involves the euthanasia of a special pet.

GRIEF

The emotional stress you experience after the loss of your pet can be overwhelming. When your dog is no longer with you, you may discover that the grieving process takes more time and more energy than you, family, or friends ever anticipated. To compound the problem of recovering from grief, our society typically does not attach as much significance to the loss of a pet as does the individual who is affected. Your loss may interfere with your daily routines, both socially and physically. Your loss may also cause old, unresolved feelings from the past to come to the surface and add to your stress and confusion. Even after you feel that you have accepted the loss, you may find that certain events or dates can temporarily cause intense feelings of loss to return.

Even though grief is an intensely personal experience and may feel like an ordeal unique to you and your situation, there are some common phases of this process that you should know to help you understand your emotions. There are different phases to the grieving process, and these phases actually help you cope with your loss. Each phase is a different length and intensity for each individual; the grieving may last for weeks, months or even years depending upon the individual and the circumstances.

The first phase you may experience after a loss is avoidance. During this phase, you may feel that the death is not real, in that it might feel as if a mistake has been made or that it is all a dream. You may experience times when you feel that the pet is in the room or nearby. These feelings can be both comforting and disturbing. Basically this phase consists of various types of denial of the situation.

The second phase of grieving is the confrontation phase, in which you realize that the death is real. During this phase, your emotions will likely be the most intense. You may experience feelings of anger, sorrow, fear, loneliness, guilt and a hodgepodge of other emotions coming and going at various times. Some people even experience a temporary questioning or loss of their faith. Feelings of guilt may arise from thinking about the things you may have failed to do for your dog, such as not going to the park more or not tending to specific health care needs. You may also feel guilty about any times you were ever angry with your dog. You may experience depression during this phase, and that depression can result in a variety of problems, such as the inability to perform daily tasks, inability to sleep, inability to get out of bed, inability to concentrate, loss of energy, exhaustion, weight loss, weight gain, and other physical symptoms. The confrontation phase may be the most confusing stage for you because of the mix of intense emotional feelings.

The last phase in the grief process is acceptance or accommodation. In this phase, the pain from the loss begins to lessen, but may not go away completely. When you reach the point of acceptance, you will find that the bittersweet memories you have of your pet are less bitter and more sweet. You will appreciate the time you shared with your pet, and you will count the joys more than the sorrows.

If you have other pets in your household, you should be aware that they are likely significantly affected by the loss. By spending more time with them, you may help them and yourself get through the emotionally difficult time a bit easier. See pages 229-230 for more information.

Pet loss support groups and grief counseling can help you understand the feelings associated with your grief, and can be valuable resources to help you through the process. Ask your veterinarian.

MEMORIALIZING

The following paragraphs should provide ideas for you to memorialize your pet. These ideas came from people who experienced the loss of a pet. You may wish to plan these activities before the loss, if possible, because after the loss you may lack the emotional energy to make decisions regarding these issues. Some of the ideas may be comforting to you, while others might not seem appropriate for you and your dog.

A memorial service with family or friends may help you acknowledge your loss. The service may be a formal gathering at a pet cemetery or may be informal and held at your home. It can be arranged with the help of the clergy, or it can be done privately. At some funerals, poetry or readings are used to honor the dog.

Special care of the remains of the dog may help memorialize the pet. A variety of options is available ranging from conventional burial and cremation to freeze drying and taxidermy. A variety of pet burial boxes and caskets is available. Some are handmade of oak and have upholstered linings, while others are not so elaborate. Special urns can be custom-made; some are made of handcarved wood while others are made of various metals. Frequently, urns have personalized engraving.

Special attention to the care of the remains may help you cope with the death. Many owners choose to place a special item in with their dog, such as its favorite blanket or toy. Some people choose to bury their dog with its collar; others choose to keep the collar for themselves. A time capsule containing photos, special toys, and/or your dog's pedigree can be buried with your dog. Some people choose to place a marker on their dog's grave, and some people replace flowers regularly at the grave site, or leave a special toy or dog treat or photograph at the grave.

Additional ideas for memorializing your pet are contained in the list that appears on the next page of this book.

ACTIVITIES TO HELP COPE WITH THE LOSS

The following is a list of activities to help cope with the loss of a special dog. Some of the activities will also serve to memorialize your dog. This list is comprised of ideas from people who have experienced the loss of a pet. Some of the ideas may be comforting to you, while others might not seem appropriate for you and your dog.

1. Plan a memorial service. See page 227.
2. Give special care to the remains. See page 227.
3. Write about your pet's life through a diary, stories or poems to document your dog's life. List the dog's favorite activities, foods, and habits.
4. Compile a photo album of your dog.
5. Collect any home videos that contain footage of your dog, and edit the clips onto one videotape of your dog.
6. Draw or paint a picture of your dog.
7. Consign an artist to paint a picture of your dog.
8. Enlarge and frame a special photo.
9. Do special activities with surviving pets.
10. Make a donation to an animal shelter or veterinary college.
11. Plant a tree in memory of your dog.
12. Join a pet loss support group
13. Call a pet loss hotline. (Ask your veterinarian or search the web.)
14. If you are ready, adopt a new pet that needs a home.

HELP FOR GRIEVING HOUSEHOLD PETS

Other pets in your household may grieve and become depressed after the loss of a special companion. Because dogs are pack animals, most dogs enjoy the company of other dogs. The loss of that instinctual bond can be debilitating for a surviving pet. Even if the surviving pet is a cat, the pet may need special attention after the loss.

Pets show grief in a variety of ways, ranging from emotional changes to physical ones. Early recognition by you of these problems may help your pet cope with the grief easier. Loss of appetite, decreased activity, and increased sleeping are common problems. Some pets obsessively search through the house for the deceased dog. Behavioral changes, such as crying, loss of house-training habits, and restlessness may also be present. Physical problems such as vomiting and diarrhea may develop. The surviving pet may be withdrawn or seek extra attention. If you note any of the above problems, seek veterinary advice to rule out a medical condition.

Your surviving pet will likely feel more secure if you spend quality time with the pet several times a day, but be careful not to encourage separation anxiety. See pages 61-65. Grooming your pet daily is also beneficial. If your pet is a dog, plan more walks. If your dog likes to ride in the car, include the pet in the trips. Help encourage eating by staying with your pet during mealtime. Provide extra toys for your pet. Leave a radio or television on for your pet to listen to while alone.

Adoption of a new pet may help prevent your pet from feeling alone, though sometimes it creates more anxiety for your pet. You are best able to judge the personality of your pet and make an educated guess as to whether a new adopted pet will help the situation.

If your pet shows signs of illness, contact your veterinarian. Similarly, if your pet does not rebound from its depression after what you feel is an adequate amount of time, contact your veterinarian.

I. Questions to Help Identify Grieving Pets

A. Note whether your surviving pet is eating after the loss.

B. Is your pet less active, sleeping more, or acting restless?

C. Does your pet search throughout the house for the dog that is gone?

D. Does your pet cry when usually it is quiet?

E. Has your pet developed any bad habits since the loss?

F. Has your pet been vomiting or does your pet have diarrhea?

G. Has your pet been withdrawn?

H. Has your pet been seeking extra attention?

If you have answered "yes' to any of these questions, your
pet may be grieving. Consult your veterinarian.

II. Suggestions for Helping Pets Cope

A. Spend additional time with your surviving pet several times a day.

B. Groom your pet daily.

C. If your pet is a dog, plan more walks.

D. If your pet likes to ride in the car, include it in the trips.

E. Stay with your pet during mealtime.

F. If there is a lack of appetite, refer to page 167-170.

G. Provide extra toys.

H. Leave a radio or television on when your pet is alone.

I. Refer any illness to a veterinarian.

J. If you are ready, adopt a new pet that needs a home.

HELP A FRIEND WHOSE DOG HAS PASSED AWAY

Friends and family can lend substantial support when a dog dies. The magnitude of the loss can be overwhelming for the owner, and support from concerned friends can be extremely helpful.

When a friend's dog passes away, make sure that you acknowledge the loss. Even if you feel somewhat awkward talking about it, or mentioning it, you should make the effort to say a few appropriate words. If you acknowledge your friend's loss, your friend will likely be appreciative of your effort. Ideally, let your friend know that he or she can talk with you about the loss. Be a good listener, and be available when your friend needs someone. Be patient; your friend may need support for a while. Offer suggestions only if necessary, such as providing a list of pet loss support groups, psychologists or clergy that may help. You may connect your friend with someone who has experienced a similar loss.

If you are invited, participate in the activities your friend arranges for memorializing the pet. If you are not invited, you may want to ask your friend whether the friend would like for you to participate. Sometimes people tend to isolate themselves during their grief, and sometimes they have difficulty asking for help.

You may wish to donate time or money, in memory of the dog, to an animal shelter or other charitable organization (e.g., the cancer society, if the dog died from cancer). The charitable organization will send an acknowledgement to the dog's owner, at your request.

A gift of food is often appropriate because it may encourage your friend to eat, even if the friend has a loss of appetite. Offering to help with a responsibility, such as baby sitting or mowing the lawn, may provide the extra assistance your friend needs if daily tasks seem to become more burdensome. An invitation to dinner or a gift certificate for dinner or a movie may encourage your friend to get out and enjoy an evening.

Remember, people grieve at different rates, and the process will take its own unique course. Being there for someone who needs to share feelings is one of the most important roles you can play in a friend's life.

APPENDICES

THE FIRST-AID KIT

A first-aid kit is important to have readily available regardless of the dog's age. The most important feature of a first-aid kit is accessibility. The kit must be available when a problem occurs. Therefore, it is important to keep the kit in a location that is obvious (e.g., beside the dog food) and in a location that provides easy access, such as an unlocked drawer or cupboard. The items in a kit should be kept within a container that is easily transported, in case you need to bring the kit to the dog. Finally, the kit should be in a closed container that will keep its contents clean and dry. A fishing tackle or utility box would be a good choice.

Once you have selected a suitable container for the kit, it is time to stock it with the items you will most likely need in an emergency. First, stock your kit with three large plastic garbage bags to protect car upholstery and household furnishings from blood, urine and feces. Then include 2 rolls of 3" gauze bandage and 12 gauze sponges 3"x3" for wound care. Obtain adhesive tape of the non-stick type; it will provide more comfort to your dog than ordinary tape that sticks to hair. Next, add scissors and toenail trimmers, several paper towels (for cleaning up messes), antibiotic ointment, saline solution (the kind people use for contact-lens cleaning), Benedryl® or diphenhydramine elixir (12.5 mg/ml liquid), tweezers, an eyedropper (for use in force-feeding liquid medications), a rectal thermometer, nonstick bandages, alcohol and hydrogen peroxide. Also include a dog muzzle, preferably the nylon variety as opposed to a leather one. A nylon muzzle is more comfortable for your pet and can be laundered easily. In a pinch you can construct a muzzle from gauze or a gentleman's necktie, but a homemade muzzle will be more difficult to use on your dog and may not work as well.

Other items that are useful but will not fit into your first-aid container should be kept in close proximity to the kit. Make sure you have two 2-liter soda bottles that you can fill with warm water in an emergency to help keep your dog from getting chilled. Also have access to clean bath towels and a blanket to aid in transportation and restraint and to provide warmth. Finally, if you have a small dog, get a pet carrier so that you can safely transport your pet in an emergency. If you have a small dog and are unable to obtain a pet carrier, make sure you have a ventilated box that is the appropriate size and is suitably durable to serve as a substitute.

To ensure you have easy access to professional help, make a list of telephone numbers of the pet's daytime veterinarian, a reserve day-time veterinarian, two night-time veterinary emergency numbers, the local poison control hotline, and the National Animal Poison Control Center. (The ASPCA Animal Poison Control Center provides assistance for a fee – $45 at the time of this printing: 1-800-548-2423.) Put one copy of the list in your first-aid kit and another near the telephone.

A copy of *Emergency First-Aid for Your Dog* (also by Dr. Tamara S. Shearer) should be kept with the kit. This book will help you respond properly in an emergency situation between the time of the emergency and the time you arrive at your veterinarian's office.

I. First-Aid Box
A. Obtain a box that is
    (1) Transportable (shoe-box size, preferably with a handle)
    (2) Durable and water-resistant (like a fishing tackle box)
    (3) Non-locking (to provide easy access).
B. Label the outside of the box "DOG FIRST AID".
C. Store the first-aid box in plain view.

II. First-Aid Provisions (to put into First-Aid Box)
A. 2 rolls of 3" gauze bandage
B. 12 gauze sponges 3"x 3"
C. Nonstick adhesive tape
D. Nonstick bandages
E. Antibiotic ointment (e.g., Polysporin®) – small tube
F. Water-soluble lubricating jelly (e.g., K-Y™ Brand)
G. Saline solution – 8 ounces (same as used for contact-lens care)
H. Hydrogen peroxide – 8 ounces
I. Alcohol
J. Eyedropper or dosage syringe
K. Tweezers
L. Scissors
M. Nail trimmers
N. Rectal thermometer

O. Muzzle – preferably nylon

P. Benedryl® or diphenhydramine elixir (12.5 mg/ml liquid)

Q. Paper towels – to clean up any mess

R. Emergency information (see below)

III. Emergency Information

A. Emergency telephone numbers:

    (1) Poison control _____

    (2) Veterinarians _____

    _____

    (3) After-hours veterinarians_____

    _____

    (4) Fire department _____

B. A copy of this book

C. A copy of the First-Aid Provisions List

D. A plant identification book

IV. Additional First-Aid Items

A. Towels – for use in restraining your dog

B. Blanket – to keep your dog warm and comfortable

C. Pet carrier – for transport if you have a dog

D. A plywood board cut to the appropriate size for your dog and for your car – to carry your injured dog safely to the car

E. Two 2-liter soda bottles – for use as hot-water bottles

MEDICAL HEALTH RECORD

Owner's Name _____

Address _____

_____

Home Phone_____ Work Phone_____

Friend/Family For Emergency Contact _____

_____

Dog's Name_____

Breed_____

Date of Birth _____

Special Diet _____

Date	Vaccination Type
_____	_____
_____	_____
_____	_____
_____	_____
_____	_____
_____	_____
_____	_____
_____	_____
_____	_____
_____	_____
_____	_____

Date	Stool Examinations & Treatment
_____	_____
_____	_____
_____	_____
_____	_____

Date	Medical Examination/Treatment/Weight
_____	_____
_____	_____
_____	_____
_____	_____
_____	_____
_____	_____

Emergency Numbers

Veterinarian_____

After-Hour Veterinarian_____

Poison Control_____

National Animal Poison Control Center_____

Fire Department_____

HOW TO MAKE AN ELIZABETHAN COLLAR

An Elizabethan collar is a cone-shaped device that fits around the dog's neck. It is used to prevent a dog from instinctively licking or chewing an external injury. Because the dog's licking or chewing can cause additional damage and promote infection, the Elizabethan collar can help prevent serious complications.

I.   **Materials Needed**
A.   Medium-weight cardboard
B.   Tape
C.   Scissors
D.   Or instead of the above items, a commercial Elizabethan collar

II. **Technique Instructions**
A.   To construct a homemade Elizabethan collar, perform the following (as illustrated on page 240):
     (1) Draw a circle on the cardboard (8 inches in diameter for a small dog with a small nose, up to 20 inches in diameter for a large dog with a large nose).
     (2) Cut out this circle.
     (3) Cut a circular hole the size of the dog's neck out of the center of the larger circle.
     (4) Make one cut from the outside diameter to the inside hole.
     (5) Slip the cardboard cut-out over the pet's head and secure the edges with tape to form a cone-like shape.
B.   Fasten the collar securely, but make sure that it does not impede the dog' breathing. It should be loose enough for you to slip two fingers under the collar. The collar should be long enough

to keep the pet from licking and chewing. It may take the dog
some time to get used to the while walking,eating and drinking.
C.   Make sure the dog will eat and drink while wearing its collar.

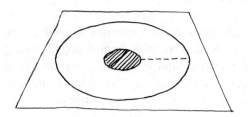

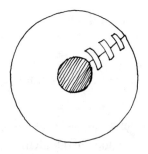

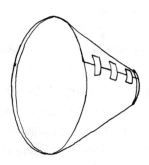

THE LOST DOG

One of the most frightening events for a dog owner is to lose a pet. Because an older dog may be confused more easily due to loss of its senses, there is an increased likelihood of getting lost. Once familiar landmarks may not be visible. The sense of smell may be diminished so the dog cannot rely on smell to find its way home. A dog with hearing loss may not be able to hear its owner calling. Proper identification will improve your chances of recovering your lost dog. If your initial attempts to locate your pet are unsuccessful, do not give up hope; many animals return home days, weeks, or months later. Even with proper identification, the dog's chances of being found can be greatly increased by following the steps described below.

I. **Information about the Lost Dog**

A. List the dog's sex, breed, color, age, name and any distinguishing characteristics.

B. Make a list of several numbers (including the veterinarian's number) for people to call if the dog is found.

C. Find a picture of the dog, if possible.

D. Decide whether to offer a reward, and if so, what amount.

II. **Daily Dog-Owner Efforts**

A. Visit shelters daily to search for the dog.
(Do not assume someone will call if the pet arrives at the shelter. Most shelters deal with hundreds of pets each day. Daily visits are important because dogs are frequently euthanized after two days if not claimed or adopted.)

B. Contact all local veterinarians by phone about the missing dog.

C. Drive through local neighborhoods calling for and asking about the dog.

D. Have neighbors help in the search. Ask them to check their garages and storage sheds.

E. Post "Lost Dog" notices. See Appendix page 243.
  (1) Include all identifying information. (See Section I above.)
  (2) Include a picture.
  (3) Indicate if there is a reward.
  (4) Use waterproof ink and sturdy paper or poster board.
  (5) Make the sign large so that it can be read from a distance.
  (6) Post signs at all major intersections within at least a 3-mile radius of the dog's home.
  (7) Post signs at local pet stores and other businesses (with their permission).
  (8) Post signs at veterinary offices.
F. Register and search on lost dog internet sites.

III. Organizations to Contact
A. Contact the local humane society.
  (1) Ask whether they have your pet.
  (2) Inquire about volunteers who run a lost and found or rescue service.
B. Contact other local shelters such as the dog/animal pound.

IV. Use of the Media
A. Run a classified advertisement for at least two weeks.
B. Check with radio and television; they often donate time during their news broadcasts to help find lost pets.

LOST PET INFORMATION

Use the following form to help find a lost dog. If your dog ever becomes lost, duplicate this form, and post it in as many locations as possible throughout the neighborhood.

LOST DOG

DESCRIPTION/BREED_____

COLOR(S)_____

SEX _____ AGE_____ WEIGHT_____ HEIGHT_____

COAT LENGTH _____

IDENTIFYING MARKS_____

TYPE AND COLOR OF COLLAR _____

LICENSE#_____ RABIES TAG#_____

AREA LOST _____

DATE LOST _____

DOG'S NAME _____

OWNER'S NAME_____

ADDRESS _____

HOME PHONE_____ WORK PHONE_____

ATTACH PICTURE HERE

NORMAL VITAL SIGNS FOR DOGS

Temperature   100 to 103 degrees Fahrenheit

Pulse/Heart Rate   100 to 130 beats per minute

Respiratory Rate   20 to 24 breaths per minute

The above signs are for a normal mature dog at rest. An excited dog, or one that has been running around, will have an elevated heart rate and an elevated respiratory rate. However, elevated vital signs for a dog at rest may be a sign of infection, disease, overheating or a variety of other health problems. Low vital signs may indicate that the dog is in shock.

BIBLIOGRAPHY

Birchard, Stephen J., D.V.M., and Robert G. Sherding, D.V.M. *Small Animal Practice.* Philadelphia: W. B. Saunders Company, 1994.

Ettinger, Stephen J., D.V.M. *Textbook of Veterinary Internal Medicine Diseases of the Dog and Cat.* 2nd ed. Philadelphia: W. B. Saunders Company, 1982.

Fenner, William R., D.V.M., ed. *Quick Reference to Veterinary Medicine.* 2nd ed. Philadelphia: J. P. Lippincott, 1991.

Fraser, Clarence M., ed. *The Merck Veterinary Manual.* 6th, 7th eds. Rathway, NJ: Merck & Co., 1986, 1991.

Goldston, Richard T., D.V.M., and Johnny D. Hoskins, D.V.M. *Geriatrics & Gerontology of the Dog and Cat.* Philadelphia: W. B. Saunders Company, 1995.

Harvey, Colin E., BVSc, FRCVS, DipACVS, DipAVDC, and Peter P. Emily, DDS, Cert Perio, Hon Men AVDC. *Small Animal Dentistry.* St. Louis: Mosby, 1993.

Kirk, Robert W., D.V.M., ed. *Current Veterinary Therapy IX: Small Animal Practice.* Philadelphia: W. B. Saunders, 1986.

Kirk, Robert W., D.V.M., and Stephen I. Bister, D.V.M. *Handbook of Veterinary Procedures and Emergency Treatment.* 4th ed. Philadelphia: W. B. Saunders, 1985.

Muller, George H., Robert W. Kirk, and Danny W. Scott. *Small Animal Dermatology.* 3rd ed. Philadelphia: W. B. Saunders, 1983.

Ogilvie, Gregory K., D.V.M., and Antony S. Moore, MVSc. *Managing the Veterinary Cancer Patient: A Practice Manual.* Ft. Collins, Colorado: Veterinary Learning Systems, 1996.

Overall, Karen L., M.A., V.M.D., Ph.D. *Clinical Behavioral Medicine for Small Animals.* St. Louis: Mosby, 1997.

Random House Webster's College Dictionary. New York: Random House, 1991.

Schoen, Allen M., D.V.M., M.S., ed. *Veterinary Acupuncture: Ancient Art of Modern Medicine.* St. Louis: Mosby, 1994.

Shearer, Tamara S., D.V.M. *Emergency First Aid For Your Dog.* Columbus, Ohio: Ohio Distinctive Publishing, 1996.

Tilley, Larry Patrick, D.V.M., Francis W. K. Smith, Jr., D.V.M., and A. Christine MacMurray, M.A. *Canine and Feline.* Baltimore: Williams & Wilkins, 1997.

INDEX

248

249

Laser surgery, 213
Last days, 221-222
Lenticular sclerosis, 66-67
Leptospirosis, 37
Lhasa Apsos, 82, 127
Lifting, 82, 135, 145, 162-165
Limping. *See* lameness, 16, 30, 32, 38, 100, 101
Listlessness 57, 77, 97
   and anemia, 54, 55
   and intestinal parasites, 126
Liver, 16, 37, 57, 130, 149
   and cancer, 30, 136
   and diarrhea, 96
   and dental disease, 87
   and heartworm, 81
   and tests, 40
   and urinary incontinence, 116, 117
   and vomiting, 146
Loss of balance. *See* Inner Ear or Vestibular Disease, 121-125
Loss of coordination, 48, 100, 118, 124
Loss of hair, 41, 84, 86, 113, 137, 141
Lost dog, 241-243
Lumps, 130-131
Lung disease. *See* Breathing Difficulties, 69-70
Lyme disease, 38, 106
Lymph nodes, 38, 130, 136
Lymphoma, 130

Magnetic resonance imaging, 42
Malignant, 42, 84, 88, 130, 136, 214
   See also Cancers
Malnutrition
   and cataracts, 66
   and diarrhea, 96
   and intestinal parasites, 126
   See also Feeding
Marking, permanent, 13-14
Massage, 176
Mast cell tumors, 130
Medical health record, 237-238
Medicines, administering, 182-185
Medicines, human, 60
Memorializing, 227
Memorial service, 227, 228
Metaclopromide, 128
Metastasis, 130
Microchip, 13
Miniature pinschers, 92
Monitoring vital signs, 179-180
Mosquitos, and heartworm, 38, 39, 81
Movement, 104, 132, 159
   restricting, 133
MRI, 42, 74, 138
Mucous in stool, 77, 96, 126, 143
Muzzle, 52, 53, 104, 234, 235

Nausea. *See* Vomiting, 146-147

Needle aspirate, 130
Nerve degeneration
   and difficulty getting up, 99-101, 161
   and hearing loss, 109
   and incontinence, 28, 61, 116, 117
Neutering, 39, 94, 137
Newfoundlands, 112
Normal vital signs for dogs, 244
Norwegian elkhounds, 127
Nuprin®. *See* ibuprofen, 57
Nutrition. *See* Feeding, 167-170
Nutritional deficiencies and anemia, 54

Obesity, 20, 62, 82, 152-153
Odor, 30, 32
Old English sheepdogs, 112, 114
Osteoporosis, 132-133
Outpatient treatment, 199

Pale or white gums, 31, 54, 69, 148
Pancreas, 40, 74, 168, 214
   and cancer, 30, 71
   and diabetes, 92
   and urinary incontinence, 116
Pancreatitis, 74, 168
Panting, 84, 141
   See also Breathing Difficulties
   See also Normal Vital Signs for Dogs
Paper training, 62, 65
Papillomas, 130
Parainfluenza, 37
Paralysis, 100, 106
Parasites
   and anemia, 54
   and colitis, 77
   and coughing, 82
   and diarrhea, 96-97
   and vomiting, 146
   and weight loss, 155
   fleas and ticks, 106-108
   intestinal, 39, 40, 61, 126
Parvovirus, 38
Pawing, 67, 88
Pekingese, 45, 82, 104
Penis, 136, 137
People food, 167, 168
Pepsid®, 128
Perianal gland tumors, 131
Peritonitis, 18
Pet loss hotlines, 220, 228
Pet loss support groups, 226, 228
Phosphorus, 40, 127, 128, 208
Physical examination. *See* Routine Preventive Health Care, 37-39
   See also Health-Care Programs
Plaque, 87-90, 193
Pneumonia, 81, 82
Poison Control Center, ASPCA Animal, 50, 235
Polyps, 88, 109, 214

250

252